COMPLETE
self
massage
WORKBOOK

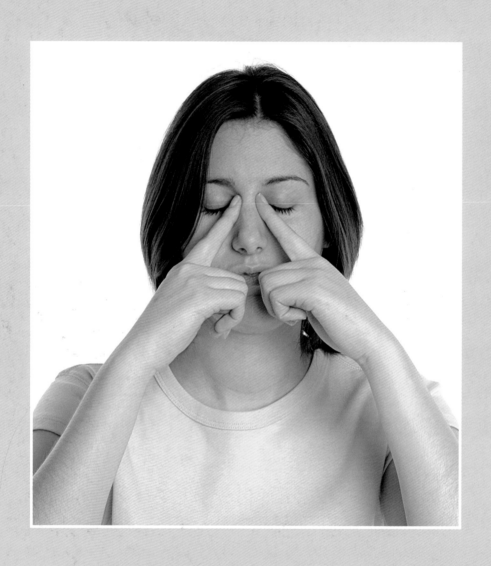

Kristine Kaoverii Weber

COMPLETE
self
massage
WORKBOOK

Over 100 Simple Techniques for
Re-energizing Body and Mind

COLLINS & BROWN

This edition published in the United Kingdom in 2015 by
Collins & Brown
1 Gower Street
London
WC1E 6HD

An imprint of Pavilion Books Company Ltd

Distributed in the United States and Canada by
Sterling Publishing Co, Inc.
387 Park Avenue South
New York
NY 10016 – 8810

ISBN 978-1-910231-38-8

A CIP catalogue record for this book is available from the British Library.

10 9 8 7 6 5 4 3 2 1

Reproduction by Classicscan, Singapore
Printed and bound by Craft Print International Ltd, Singapore

This book can be ordered direct from the publisher at www.pavilionbooks.com
Front cover photography: Shutterstock
Photography by Neil Sutherland

Safety Note
The information in this book is not intended as a substitute for medical advice.
Any person suffering from conditions requiring medical attention, or who has
symptoms that concern them, should consult a qualified medical practitioner.

Contents

Introduction

Before there were muscle-relaxants, aspirins or chiropractors, people used their hands to rub away their aches and pains. Massage is the most basic healing tool, and human beings have long recognized its curative power. We know massage has a long and well-respected history because the art and literature of many ancient cultures, from China and India to Greece and Egypt, depict massage as an integral part of their healing systems. In modern times, in the Western world, massage was not considered a serious healing method until the latter part of the twentieth century. Today massage is enjoying a renaissance, and its popularity is growing as the styles of massage therapy become more varied and sophisticated. Many people now consider regular professional massage essential to their physical – as well as their mental and emotional – well-being.

Having selected this book, you may be well aware of the benefits of massage and may have experienced some of them first hand. You may be familiar with the special power of self-massage, which is a natural way to take care of ourselves, and we instinctively understand its potential. When we injure ourselves, our first reaction is to hold and soothe a stubbed toe or a bumped elbow. When we have a headache, we hold our forehead or rub the back of our neck; and strained eyes welcome the soothing pressure of warm fingertips.

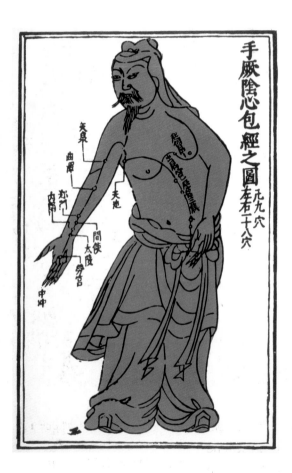

An ancient Chinese illustration of acupuncture zones.

Even the simplest self-massage techniques can confer a wide range of benefits, ranging from relaxation and stress relief to improving circulation and reducing pain. Specific, powerful techniques will help to alleviate a variety of symptoms, with even greater results. This book will serve as your guide to the healing world of self-massage.

All the techniques in this book are simple and clearly illustrated, so they are easy to understand and perform. Many of them can be done just about anywhere: at the office or on

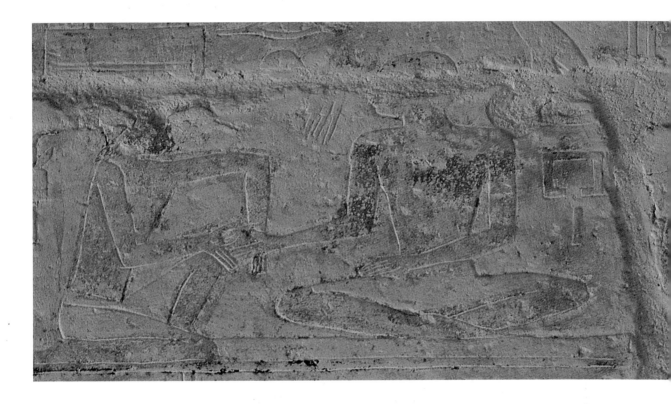

an aeroplane – even during a business meeting. Some self-massage is best practised when you can find some quiet time to relax afterwards, but the "quick fix" massages can help, even when you're on the go. You can choose the massage technique that best fits your situation and lifestyle.

This book is not intended to replace medical care, or cure any illness. If you have any serious health conditions, check with your doctor before using this guide to self-massage.

An Ancient Egyptian wall painting from the tomb of Ankhmahor, circa 2345 to 2181 BC. The scene depicts a hand massage being given.

How to use this book

You have probably picked up this book because you have an intuitive understanding of the healing power in your hands. The information here will give you a framework through which you can harness that energy, in order to assuage the minor discomforts of modern life and feel better in general. Share what you learn with your friends and family so that they too can experience their own innate healing ability.

PART 1: MASSAGE TECHNIQUES

This section will familiarize you with the various techniques necessary to perform self-massage safely and effectively. You will notice that massage techniques vary widely. While Swedish techniques are long and soothing, acupressure techniques are more focused. Reflexology uses different techniques again, with direct but moving pressure on a particular point. You certainly don't have to become an expert to use these self-massage techniques effectively, but having some familiarity with the different styles will help you implement the exercises given in this book with greater confidence and success.

PART 2: DIRECTORY OF EVERYDAY CONDITIONS

Each condition generally has two or three different techniques to help you address your discomfort, based on your specific situation. Some entries include "quick fix" help, which may be more appropriate when you are at the office or pressed for time. However, the majority of the techniques will take you no more than 15 minutes, and many of them can be performed discreetly in just about any setting. Remember that consistency is important, and that following the recommended guidelines on how many times a day you should perform the massage will make your self-treatment more successful. If one technique does not work for you, attempt another and see if you get better results. Always try to make yourself as comfortable as possible while performing these massages. Relax and breathe deeply. Being relaxed is important while performing self-massage because it activates a deeper response. This natural healing response is an essential element of successful self-treatment.

PART 3: WELLNESS ROUTINE

This section introduces you to "do-in", the ancient Chinese method of self-massage. This is an excellent treatment for general well-being and relaxation. Using this massage on a daily basis can keep you energized and in good health.

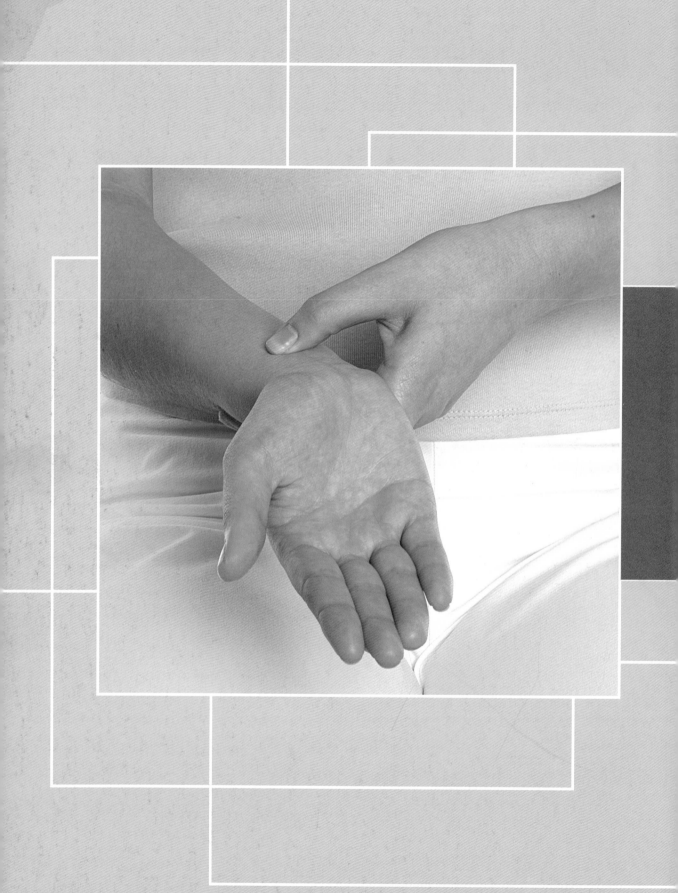

MASSAGE TECHNIQUES

Swedish/classic massage

The origins

Swedish or classic massage is the most widely recognized form of massage therapy available today – and the most popular. Its origins are generally attributed to Dr Per Henrik Ling (1776–1839), a fencer who developed a rheumatic condition in his shoulder and cured himself with a combination of exercise and massage. He then promoted his system of cure, which became known as the "Swedish Movement Treatment".

Ling's system was unique in that it combined some form of exercise with the massage of a specific area. Clearly, Ling contributed to popularizing massage as a form of therapy. However, the basic Swedish massage strokes that are taught and used today were created by a Dutch practitioner named Johan Georg Mezger (1838–1909). He adopted the French names to label the basic strokes under which he systematized his specific type of therapy, which later became known as Swedish or classic massage.

Swedish massage forms the basis of just about all other Western-style massage. Having some familiarity with Swedish strokes is essential in practising effective self-massage.

How does it work?

Swedish massage relies on several primary strokes, which are used in variation. Each type of stroke is thought to have a specific therapeutic effect. These include the relaxation of muscles and localized areas of knottiness, increasing blood and lymphatic circulation, the relief of pain and helping the body to recover from muscle strain. The strokes are generally directed towards the heart, as this assists circulation and helps process the toxins that are released from muscles during massage. However, for self-massage this is not always practical – for example, in the foot massage (see *page 14*), you will be stroking away from the heart. Swedish self-massage is contraindicated in cases of skin infection, wounds, incisions, bruises and inflammation.

The strokes

Although there are several different kinds of Swedish massage technique, the following three will give you enough skill to practise basic self-massage. Don't worry about remembering the French names of the techniques, since all of the massages in this book use the English translation.

The strokes

Long stroking (effleurage)

This stroke is the most commonly used technique in Swedish massage. It is a simple gliding action over the skin.

Kneading (petrissage)

This is a kneading stroke used to lift up the muscle and wring or squeeze it. Petrissage is used to rid the muscle of waste and break up adhesions.

Friction

Friction is often used go a little deeper into the muscle than stroking or kneading. It is good for using on small areas of the body and around bones.

Practising a Swedish foot massage on yourself

To practise effleurage on yourself, take off your socks, sit in a comfortable chair and place your left foot over your right thigh. (If you are not flexible enough to do this, don't worry — another technique will be given later, which will enable you to practise effleurage.) Rub your hands together to warm them. If you like, you can use a small amount of natural vegetable oil, but this is not essential.

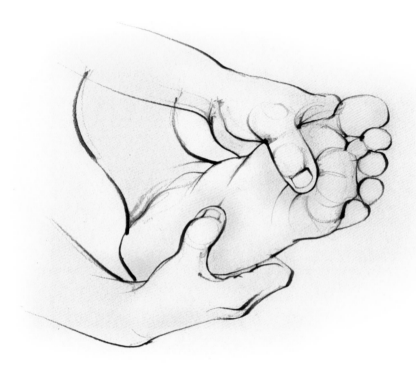

Using your thumbs, slide the whole inside of one thumb up the sole of the foot, from the heel to the toes. Before you finish this first stroke, follow with your other thumb in the same way. Use extra pressure in sore areas. Shorten the stroke to attend to specific points. Continue this thumb-over-thumb stroking for about two minutes, and then repeat on the other foot.

Practising a Swedish arm massage on yourself

If you can't reach your feet comfortably and easily, try effleurage on your arms. You may want to wear a short-sleeved T-shirt for this practice. Rub your hands together to warm them. If you like, you can use a small amount of natural vegetable oil, but this is not essential.

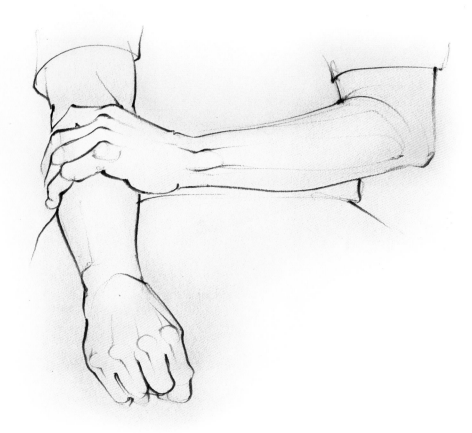

1 Place your hand over your wrist, with the fingers curled around the outside of your wrist and your thumb tucked under the wrist. Keep your fingers together. With a little pressure, slide (in one stroke) up the arm to the shoulder. Repeat this several times.

2 Next, sit still for a few moments and compare the sensations in your arms. You may notice a warm, tingling or relaxed feeling in the arm you have massaged. Repeat the same technique on your other arm.

Practising a Swedish shoulder massage on yourself

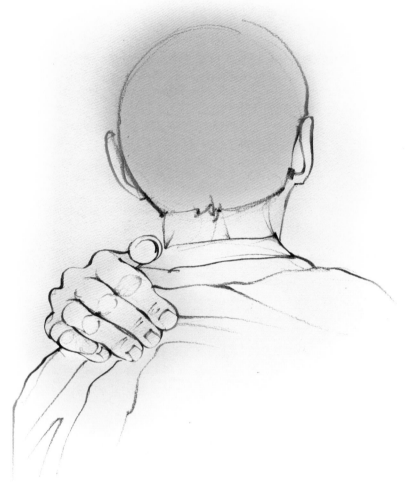

1 Sit in a comfortable chair. Use long, deep strokes on your left shoulder, by sliding the fingers of your right hand from the base of your skull to the outside of your shoulder a few times. Keep the fingers together.

2 For kneading (petrissage) place your fingers and thumb together at the back of the thick muscle band on top of your shoulder. Let the heel of your hand rest just above your collar bone. Now squeeze your fingers and the heel of your hand together and hold briefly. Repeat this action

several times. Move your hand to a slightly different spot after each squeeze. You can spend more time on, and press more deeply into, sore spots. Continue for at least one minute.

3 Now sit still, take a few deep breaths and notice the difference in feeling between your shoulders. Repeat on the other shoulder. Vary the pressure you apply by sometimes pressing your fingertips more deeply into any tight muscle area and sometimes pressing hard with the heel of your hand.

Practising a Swedish jaw massage on yourself

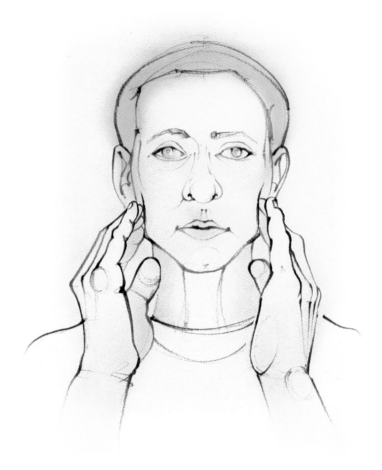

1 Place your fingertips on your cheeks in front of your ears. Clench your jaws together and you will feel a muscle pop out – this is the muscle you will practise on. Relax your jaw and begin to make small circular motions with your fingertips into this muscle, circling in both directions. This stroke, unsurprisingly, is called "circular friction". The area may feel sore, so start gently and slowly increase the pressure. Continue for about one minute.

2 Next, experiment by moving your fingertips to different areas of the muscle, again making small circular motions. Continue for another minute. This muscle is often very tight and has many small knots, which you may begin to feel as you massage the area. This simple self-massage, when used daily, can lessen tension of the jaw.

Acupressure

The origins

Acupressure is a general term which describes any type of massage that stimulates acupoints (pressure points) on the body in an attempt to achieve a therapeutic effect. It originated in Asia and has been an important part of Chinese medicine for thousands of years. In the twentieth century acupressure spread throughout the world and transformed itself into a variety of different styles. Some of the styles that are popular today include jin shin jitsu, shiatsu, zen shiatsu, shen tao, jin shen, jin shin do, tuina, acu-yoga and do-in (see *pages 86–93*). All forms of acupressure use finger, hand, elbow or foot pressure on the various acupoints. Some combine massage techniques, while others are strictly point-focused; some use strong pressure, while others apply very light pressure. The acupressure self-help guidelines in this book are simple and straightforward to enable you to achieve great results.

Meridians

Acupressure uses specific points that lie on "meridians" or "channels". These invisible lines carry "chi", or life-force energy, throughout the body. The 12 main meridians are controlled by different organs – for example, the liver, kidneys or heart. If you imagine the meridians as rivers of energy, then the acupoints are like small pools or dams in those rivers. Sometimes the pools get too full and at other times they are too empty. Applying pressure can regulate the flow so that these rivers run more smoothly.

Chinese medical theory

Chinese medicine is a sophisticated and ancient system, which has been in existence for more than 5,000 years. Chinese medical practitioners use various diagnostic tools, such as the condition of the tongue and the quality of 12 different pulses on the wrist, to determine the course of treatment for each individual. Treatment may include acupuncture, herbs, moxa (a warming herb that is placed on the outside of the body and burned), cupping (the use of suction on certain acupoints), acupressure and massage. Although this complex system of medicine takes years to master, simple and safe acupressure techniques can be practised by just about anyone. Familiarizing yourself with a few basic techniques can help you cope with minor ailments and maintain your health.

How do I perform acupressure?

You can visualize acupoints as being about the size of the pad of your thumb, or even a little larger. You don't have to be tremendously precise in finding the points; however, noticing a soreness or nervy sensation as you are feeling for the acupoint will help you locate it more accurately and treat it more effectively. Some points are more sensitive than others, and occasionally you won't have any soreness at the location. In this case, if you have carefully followed the instructions, you should trust that you have located the point correctly. Once you find the acupoint, steady, sustained pressure or small circular massage strokes (usually for about one to three minutes) is often sufficient stimulation. It is generally important to stimulate the same point on both sides of the body if possible.

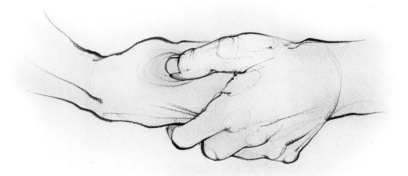

Stimulating the acupoint Large Intestine 4 or "hoku" point, which is one of the most well-known points and is commonly used for conditions such as headaches, tooth pain and constipation.

19

Reflexology techniques

The origins

Reflexology is the application of pressure to points on the hands or feet, which correspond to certain parts of the body. Although it is commonly believed that reflexology came from China, there is evidence that it was also used in Ancient Egyptian, Babylonian and Native North American cultures. A carving at a physician's tomb in Saqquara in Egypt (dating to 2350 BC) depicts what looks like both a foot and hand reflexology treatment.

The longitudinal zones

The reflexology used in the West today has its origin in nineteenth-century Russian and Germany scientific enquiry. An American, Dr William Fitzgerald, who studied reflex theory while working in Vienna, consolidated some of this research along with his own theories and published the book *Zone Therapy* in 1917.

Fitzgerald divided the body into 10 equal longitudinal zones of energy, running from the feet, up the legs, down the arms and up into the brain. The zones were numbered from one to five, from the middle of the body to the outside, on both sides. Fitzgerald theorized that any impairment to the free flow of life-force energy or chi, would affect the vital parts of the body and the organs within that specific zone.

Reflex zones of the foot

Fitzgerald taught zone therapy to a friend and colleague, Dr Shelby Riley. However, it was Riley's associate, Eunice Ingham, a physical therapist, who became particularly enthusiastic about the work. Ingham experimented with the effects of working on different areas of the feet in relation to the 10 longitudinal zones, until she was able to map the entire body on the feet.

Practising reflexology techniques

Because the reflex areas are minute, they must be stimulated directly and precisely. Circular friction-massage or back-and-forth rubbing is not as effective as pinching an area, rotating on a point or thumb-walking.

PINCHING

Pinching is exactly what it sounds like – you pinch with your index finger and thumb to precisely stimulate an area. The thumb is usually the tool that stimulates the reflex zone, while the index finger stabilizes the thumb on the other side of the hand or foot.

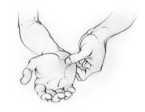

1 *Pinching*

ROTATING ON A POINT

For this technique, place your thumb on the reflex zone and your other fingers around the back of the foot or hand. Press into the area with your thumb, supporting the pressure with your fingers from the other side. Then rotate your thumb as you continue to hold the pressure.

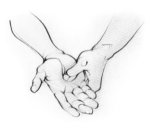

2 *Rotating on a point*

THUMB-WALKING

This technique may take a little more practice. It is often described as using the thumb to crawl like a caterpillar over the reflex zone. Place the pad of your thumb on your opposite palm. Now bend the knuckle so that you roll up to the tip of your thumb (see 3a).

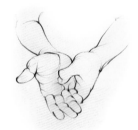

3a *Thumb-walking*

Next, flatten your thumb again, but move it forward about 0.5 cm (¹/₄ inch). Never let your thumb lose contact with the skin (see 3b). Repeat the action over your palm several times until it becomes an easy repetitive action.

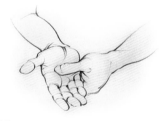

3b

Other massage techniques

Other styles of massage suggested in this book include trigger-point therapy, Indian head massage, manual lymphatic drainage and aromatherapy massage – all of which use simple massage techniques. If you follow the instructions carefully, you will have no difficulty in implementing any of the techniques.

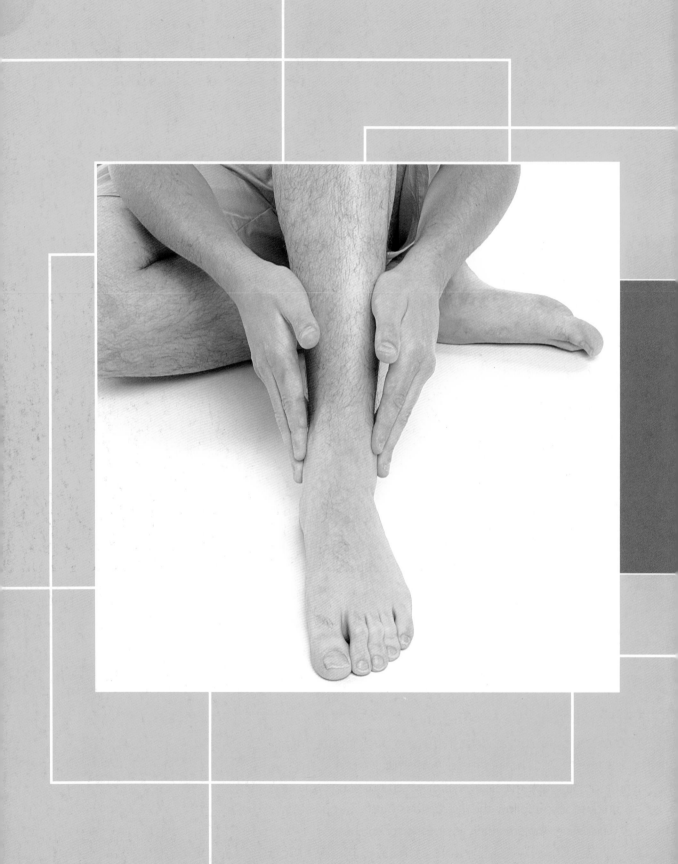

DIRECTORY OF EVERYDAY CONDITIONS

2

Anxiety

For some people, situations such as being interviewed for a job or giving a speech can be paralysing. Self-massage can help to reduce anxiety and make these everyday situations easier to cope with. While chronic anxiety should always be addressed by a health professional, the techniques given below may both alleviate everyday anxiety and complement a professional approach to more serious anxiety issues.

Self-massage help

AIMS
to loosen up the muscles involved in breathing and help relieve anxiety

FREQUENCY
twice a day

CONTRAINDICATIONS
any chronic lung or heart condition

CROSS-REFERENCE
Breathing issues p. 30

Anxiety creates mental and emotional tension, as well as difficulty in breathing and an increased heart rate. Massaging the chest can help to relieve muscular tension, make breathing easier and alleviate the emotional component of anxiety.

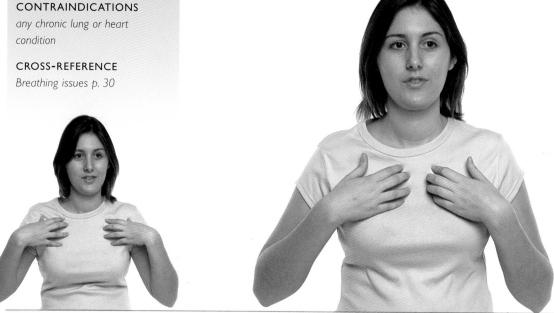

1 *With your fingers separated, massage the muscles between the ribs with your fingertips. Start at the outer part of your chest just under the collarbone and massage towards the heart.*

2 *Move your fingertips to the ribs in front of the armpits and continue massaging. Massage towards the sternum (breastbone), first from the armpit to the area outside the nipple and then from the area inside the nipple to the sternum.*

Here are some other tips to help you cope with anxiety-producing situations:
- Get regular cardiovascular exercise and plenty of sleep.
- Cut down on caffeine consumption or cut it out altogether.
- Instead of reaching for cigarettes to quell anxiety, find a gentle yoga class and attend several days a week.
- Adding a few drops of lavender essential oil to a warm bath or to oil for a foot massage (*see pages 80–81*) can help.
- Consider scheduling a professional massage the day before a particularly anxiety-producing event, such as a public lecture or business meeting.

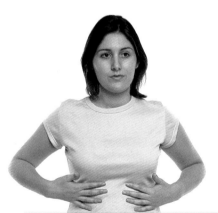

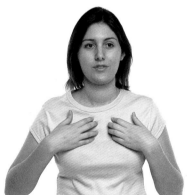

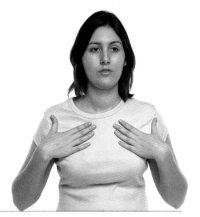

3 *Place your fingertips below your breast tissue and massage the lower ribs, from the sides of the body towards the bottom of the sternum.*

4 *Next, take a deep breath. As you are breathing in, tap around the whole ribcage with your fingertips.*

5 *As you exhale, slap your chest and lower ribs with the palms of your hands. Repeat steps 4 and 5 for three to four deep breaths.*

Acupressure help

AIMS
to calm the mind and body

FREQUENCY
several times a day, as needed

CONTRAINDICATIONS
none known

CROSS-REFERENCE
Menstrual discomfort p. 60

ALSO BENEFICIAL FOR
P 8 – fatigue, hardening of the arteries, high blood pressure
P 6 – nausea, morning and motion sickness, vomiting, insomnia, palpitations, epilepsy

The hands have several acupoints that are useful for helping to calm the mind. In old movies, when something goes wrong there is often a scene in which the heroine is found "wringing her hands". This hand-massaging is actually an instinctive way of coping with stress. Massaging the hands is very soothing and can help to diminish anxiety.

The Pericardium meridian, which runs straight down the middle of the inside of the arm, is particularly important in treating anxiety and stress. The pericardium itself is the sheath or covering which protects the heart. In terms of Chinese medicine, which is more metaphorical and poetic than western medicine, this "protection" is not only physical, it is emotional as well.

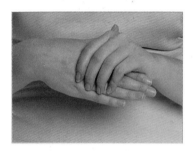

1 *Slowly and completely massage your hands, fingers and wrists. Pay attention to any sore areas and give them some extra time.*

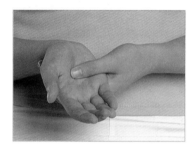

2 *Massage Pericardium 8: place your thumb in the centre of the palm and massage in circles for about one minute. Repeat on the other hand.*

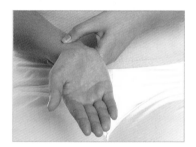

3 *Massage Pericardium 6: place your thumb in between the tendons on the inside of the wrist. Slide up about two-and-a-half finger widths. Massage in circles for about one minute. Repeat on the other wrist.*

Chakra-balancing self-help

AIMS
to calm the mind and body

FREQUENCY
several times a day, as needed

CONTRAINDICATIONS
none known

ALSO BENEFICIAL FOR
centring, grounding and focusing attention

This self-massage is used to balance the chakras. Eastern medicine believes that there are major energy centres (chakras) in seven main places along the spine, which resonate out through both the front and back of the body. Imbalances in the chakras lead to mental/emotional imbalances. In this massage, visualize using the calming, healing energy of your hands to balance the chakras. Both the fourth and sixth chakras contain acupoints that are beneficial for anxiety. After completing the following exercise, you can use your fingertips to do small circular massage on each area.

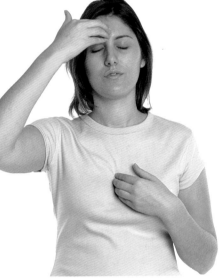

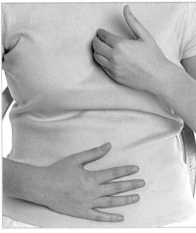

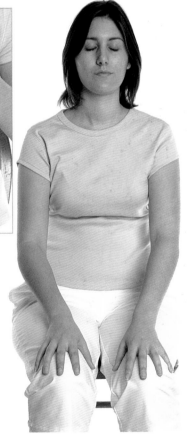

1 *Close your eyes and place the fingertips of one hand in the centre of the sixth chakra (between the eyebrows) and the fingertips of your other hand in the centre of the fourth chakra (in the middle of the chest). Breathe deeply and feel a connection between your hands.*

2 *After several deep breaths, remove your fingers from the sixth chakra and place that hand over your stomach at the navel. Let your breath and attention move down your body. Imagine that your anxiety is melting away and pouring down into the earth.*

3 *Next, rest both hands in your lap for a few deep breaths before opening your eyes.*

Arthritis

Self-massage can provide great relief for people suffering from arthritis. Because there are so many different kinds of arthritis, certain techniques will work better for some people than for others. Try a few to see which technique is right for you. Do not massage inflamed joints directly, because massage can actually make inflammation worse. If your symptoms are flaring up, it is best to use acupoints away from the site of the arthritis and to massage around, but not directly on, the joint. Here are some self-massage suggestions for specific arthritis issues.

Self-massage for hand pain

AIMS
to ease sore and aching joints in the hands

FREQUENCY
five-minute massage once or twice a day

CONTRAINDICATIONS
inflamed joints

CROSS-REFERENCE
Joint mobility p. 52

ALSO BENEFICIAL FOR:
overworked hands

When your symptoms are not active, daily self-massage to the area where you have arthritis can be very helpful. It is important to emphasize range of motion in the joints. For range of motion, support around the joint with one or both hands (here we are massaging the finger so you can only use one hand, but on an ankle or toe, you should use two). Move the joint gently in all directions. If you feel pain, you are stretching the joint too far.

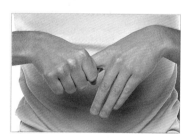
1 Massage the joints that are most arthritic. Rotate each finger; bend and stretch each finger.

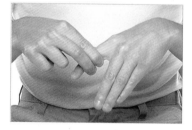
2 Massage the bones around the joint. Slide your fingers up and down and squeeze each bone several times. This will massage the nerves that feed into the painful joint.

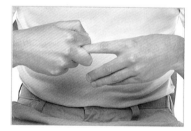
3 Squeeze the tip of each finger and then quickly pull your hand off the end to stimulate blood flow.

Acupressure self-help for hand pain

AIMS
to ease sore and aching joints in the hands

FREQUENCY
several times a day

CONTRAINDICATIONS
pregnancy

CROSS-REFERENCE
Headaches p. 46, Joint mobility p. 52, Toothache p. 82

ALSO BENEFICIAL FOR
constipation, headache, toothache, facial pain, colds

This acupoint is excellent for many types of pain. For the best results, use it in addition to the self-massage for hand pain given opposite.

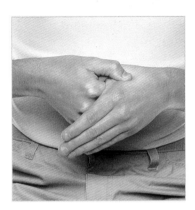

Press Large Intestine 4: to find this point, slide your thumb down to the point where the bones of the thumb and index finger meet, then turn your thumb up and press into the index finger bone. You will feel a "zingy" or nervy sensation. Massage the point in small circles for one to two minutes.

Acupressure self-help for knee pain

AIMS
to relieve knee pain, especially arthritic pain

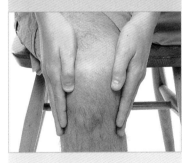

FREQUENCY
two to three times a day

CONTRAINDICATIONS
none known

CROSS-REFERENCE
Knee pain p. 54

ALSO BENEFICIAL FOR
constipation, stomach problems, fatigue

This massage will prove to be especially beneficial if you can practise it at least once a day.

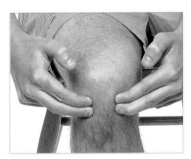

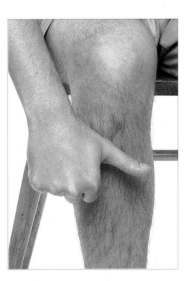

Begin by briskly rubbing the knee between both palms. Massage the muscles around the knee. Continue for two to three minutes.

2 Massage acupoint "Xiyan", located on both sides of the tendon just below the kneecap, with your index and middle fingers, for one to two minutes.

3 Next, use the knuckles to rub Stomach 36, located about four finger widths below the outside of the kneecap, for one to two minutes.

Breathing issues

You can use self-massage techniques to help calm the body so that breathing is more comfortable. The massages shown here will help to strengthen and revitalize the lung and kidney chi and can make breathing a little easier. While self-massage techniques will not cure breathing issues, they can complement medical care and act as tools to enable you to take an active role in your own healing process.

Self-massage help

AIMS
to help improve breathing

FREQUENCY
two to three times a day

CONTRAINDICATIONS
for serious breathing conditions, such as Chronic Obstructive Pulmonary Disease (COPD), always check with your doctor first

CROSS-REFERENCE
Anxiety p. 24

Poor posture and shallow breathing can inhibit the chest muscles and compromise breathing capacity. This self-massage technique will help to release tension in the chest and free up the muscles used in breathing.

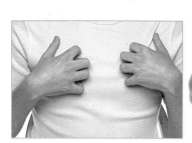

1 *Quickly tap the upper front ribs with your fingertips as you take a deep breath.*

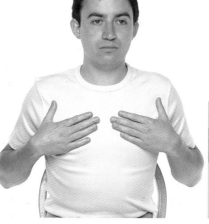

2 *Exhale through your mouth and repeatedly slap the upper ribs using your whole palm. Repeat steps 1 and 2 three times. Repeat the whole process three times on the lower front ribs.*

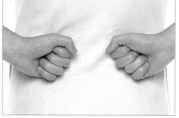

3 *Make fists with your hands and massage the kidney area, located just under the ribs in the back, with your knuckles. Massage for about one minute.*

Acupressure self-help

AIMS
to ease colds, coughs, asthma, bronchitis and fever

FREQUENCY
two to three times a day

CONTRAINDICATIONS
none known

CROSS-REFERENCE
Neck and shoulder tension p. 66

ALSO BENEFICIAL FOR
shoulder and upper back pain caused by respiratory issues

For a cold or cough, practise this massage a few times a day. Do not be concerned about finding acupoints precisely. In acupressure, we can think about points being as large as a medium-sized coin. Even if your point location is a little off, the massage itself is relaxing and will help. This massage can also be helpful for chronic breathing problems.

If you have time, combine this treatment with the self-massage help shown opposite to create better results.

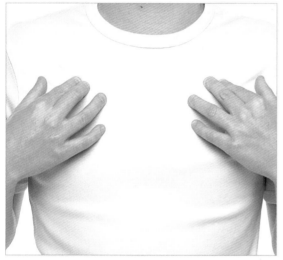

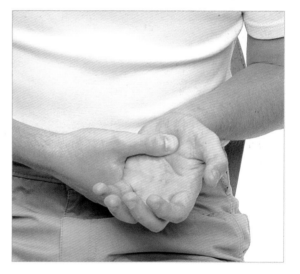

I *In the space beneath the collarbone on both sides of the body, where the collar bone meets the shoulder, you will find a soft area that may feel tender as you press in with your fingers. This is the general area of acupoints Lung 1 and 2, which are excellent points to help free up the lungs and make breathing easier. Place two or more fingers in this soft area and massage in gentle circles for at least one minute.*

2 *Next, find the acupoint Lung 10, which is located in the centre of the pad of the thumb. This excellent acupoint is also great for freeing up the breath. It is easy to find because it often feels a bit tender. Massage this point on both hands for at least one minute each.*

Circulation issues

There are many causes of poor circulation, some of them more serious than others. If your circulation has recently become poor, it is essential that you consult a doctor, determine the reason and treat the condition appropriately. Some of the causes of poor circulation include diabetes, arteriosclerosis (hardening of the arteries), Raynaud's disease, smoking, high blood pressure, high cholesterol, obesity, varicose veins and phlebitis (inflammation of the veins). But poor circulation may also simply be a case of prolonged exposure to cold or lack of exercise, or may be caused by hereditary factors. Whatever the cause, massage is generally a way to help improve circulation. If you have a serious circulatory problem, consult your doctor before trying these self-help techniques.

Self-massage help

AIMS
to improve the circulation in general, specifically to the hands and feet

FREQUENCY
twice a day

CONTRAINDICATIONS
foot ulcers or any other open wounds

CROSS-REFERENCE
Joint mobility p. 52, Tired feet p. 80

ALSO BENEFICIAL FOR
calming the mind, grounding

Massage is an excellent way to improve the circulation. In fact, improved circulation is one of the most widely touted health benefits of massage. For more detailed instructions on these massages, see the cross-references listed opposite.

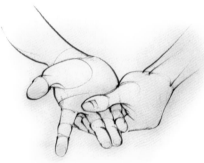 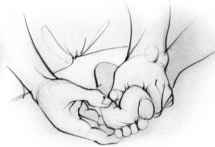

1 *Use quick, strong strokes to completely massage your hands, fingers and wrists. Pay particular attention to any sore areas, giving them some extra time. You may want to use massage oil or cream.*

2 *Apply massage oil or cream to your feet. Use quick, strong strokes to completely massage your feet, toes and ankles. Again, pay particular attention to any sore areas.*

Reflexology self-help

AIMS
*to improve the circulation in
general, specifically to the hands
and feet*

FREQUENCY
twice a day

CONTRAINDICATIONS
*open wounds, foot ulcers in the
reflex zone*

CROSS-REFERENCE
Energy-boosters p. 40

ALSO BENEFICIAL FOR
fatigue

*With your foot placed on your
opposite thigh, trace a line
straight down towards your ankle
from the inside of the big toe. The
adrenal reflex zone is a little less
than halfway down (see right)
Use thumb-walking (see page 21)
on this area. Continue for two
minutes, then repeat on the
other foot.*

Massaging the adrenal reflex area of the feet can help to improve circulation. This reflex area may seem difficult to locate, but it is generally sore, tender or tight on most people (because most of us ask a lot of our adrenal glands!)

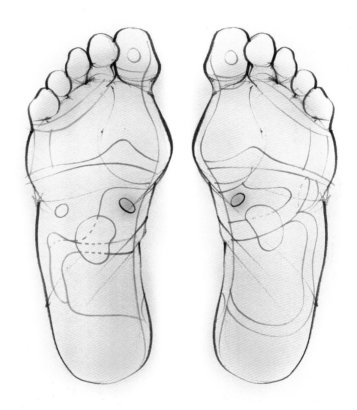

Computer strain

If you spend a lot of time at the computer, you will know that even though you are sitting still, your body takes a beating. Having an ergonomically correct workspace can ease the strain of intense computer work. Your feet should be flat on the floor, your lower back supported, the screen should be at eye level and your wrists and forearms straight. Look away from the screen frequently and get up and take a break every hour. Even if you follow these guidelines, you still may suffer from tired eyes, sore wrists or carpal tunnel syndrome, a painful lower back, and aching shoulders and neck. However, self-massage can help.

Self-massage help

AIMS
to relieve the strain caused by computer use

FREQUENCY
five-minute routine, three to four times a day

CROSS-REFERENCE
*Circulation issues p. 32,
Eye strain p. 42, Joint mobility
p. 52, Low backache p. 56,
Neck and shoulder tension p. 66*

ALSO BENEFICIAL FOR
other types of repetitive strain activity

Here is a quick routine that you can use during a work break to help heal your body from the overall strain of sitting for long hours at the computer. If you have a specific ailment from using your computer (for example, lower back pain), use the cross-references to help you find a more extensive massage for the part of the body in question.

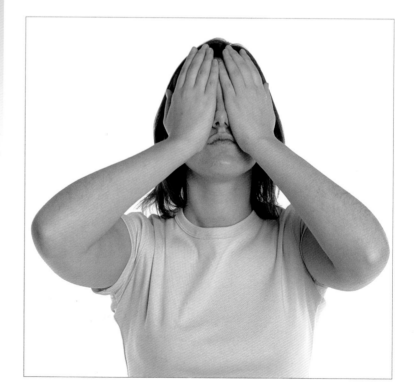

Begin by rubbing your hands together to warm them. Place your warm palms over your eyes and take two deep breaths. Repeat two to three times.

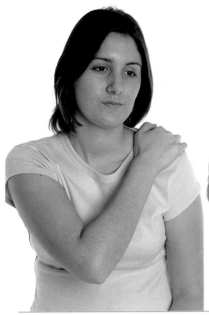

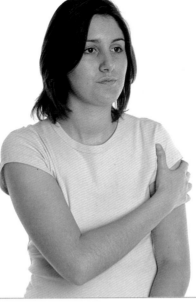

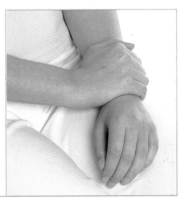

2 Use your right hand to knead your left shoulder.

3 Next, knead your upper arm, and continue this action down to your wrist and hand.

Repeat two to three times. Spend some extra time squeezing your wrist.

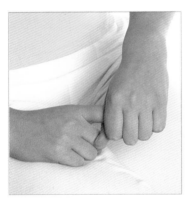

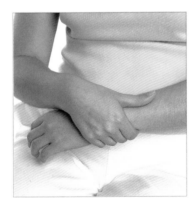

Use the same action on the inside of your forearm. Repeat the whole sequence on the right side. Finally, make fists with your hands. Lean forward and vigorously rub the lower back with your knuckles, up and down and from side to side. Continue for at least one minute.

4 Now squeeze and twist each finger in turn.

5 Place your right thumb in the centre of your outer wrist crease. With deep pressure, stroke your thumb up your forearm about one-third of the way to your elbow. Repeat this stroke several times.

Constipation

If constipation is a chronic problem for you, try one of these routines daily for a week or two and you may see some significant results. One technique may work better than another or be more convenient for your lifestyle. Constipation should also be addressed by reassessing your diet and making the appropriate changes. For example, you may need to add more fibre and decrease your intake of refined foods. The following self-massage techniques can be helpful for chronic as well as occasional constipation.

Self-massage help

AIMS
to improve the peristaltic action of the large intestine

In addition to helping ease the occasional bout of constipation, this simple self-massage will soothe and strengthen your digestive system.

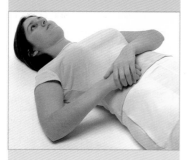

FREQUENCY
daily for chronic conditions; several times a day for occasional constipation

CONTRAINDICATIONS
any serious abdominal injury, surgery or tumours

CROSS-REFERENCE
Indigestion p. 50

ALSO BENEFICIAL FOR
soothing an upset stomach

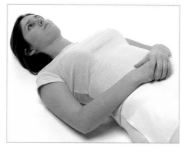

1 *Sit on a chair or lie on the floor. Make a fist with your right hand and place it on the right side of your abdomen. Clasp your right hand with your left hand (left).*

2 *Breathe in. As you exhale, press down with your hands and slide them around your abdomen in a large, clockwise circle. Complete the circle as you finish one full, slow exhalation. Repeat this step 10 times.*

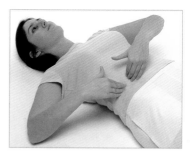

3 *Next, imagine that you have a large clock on your abdomen. Use all of your fingertips together to massage each "hour" of the clock with small, clockwise circular pressure. Start on your right side (at about nine o'clock, if 12 o'clock is just under your breastbone) and work your way around in a circle. Massage each hour of the clock for about 15 seconds. Make two complete rounds.*

Acupressure quick fix

AIMS
to relieve constipation

FREQUENCY
several times a day

CONTRAINDICATIONS
pregnancy

CROSS-REFERENCE
Arthritis p. 28, Toothache p. 82

ALSO BENEFICIAL FOR
diarrhoea, rashes, tooth and facial pain

One of the most powerful and well-known acupoints, Large Intestine 4, has a variety of applications. It is an easy-to-access acupoint that you can use at any time.

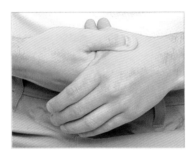

1 *Find Large Intestine 4, located on the back of the hand, in the web between the thumb and index finger. To access the point most effectively, slide your thumb to the place where the index finger and thumb bones meet, then press into the index finger bone. You will probably feel a "zingy" or nervy sensation when you find the point. Press and hold for one minute, or massage in small circles. Massage this point using circular pressure for about one minute. Repeat on the other hand.*

2 *Massage from the tip of your index finger down a straight line back to Large Intestine 4. This is the beginning of the Large Intestine meridian. Massaging this line encourages the flow of energy in the right direction and can help alleviate constipation. Repeat on your other hand.*

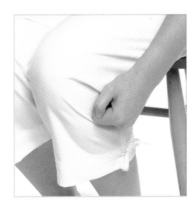

3 *Now, place your knuckles on Stomach 36 on both legs, located just below the kneecap on the outside of the shinbone. Rub this area with your knuckles briskly for about one minute.*

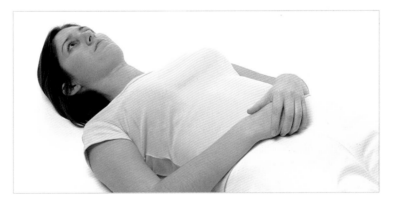

4 *Next, place your fist just between your pubic bone and navel, and gently press into your stomach. Use your whole fist to massage the area of Conception Vessel 6 – a commonly used acupoint for constipation.*

Reflexology self-help

AIMS
to relieve constipation

FREQUENCY
twice a day

CONTRAINDICATIONS
colitis, irritable bowel syndrome

ALSO BENEFICIAL FOR
diarrhoea

The colon reflex zone on the feet starts at the bottom of the right foot and moves over to the left foot (see below) Following this sequence exactly allows you to trace the path of the large intestine and help to improve the flow of energy through this part of your body. Note that if you have diarrhoea, you should treat in the opposite direction to reverse the energy flow.

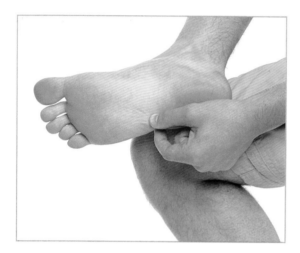

Use your left thumb to work on the bottom of your right foot. Thumb-walk (see page 21) towards the little toe in the reflex zone, as shown here.

2 *Next, thumb-walk across the centre of your right foot.*

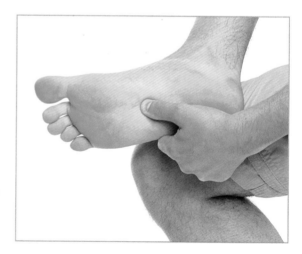

3 *Switch feet. Use your left thumb to work the bottom of your left foot. Thumb-walk across the centre of your left foot, from the inside of the arch to the outside.*

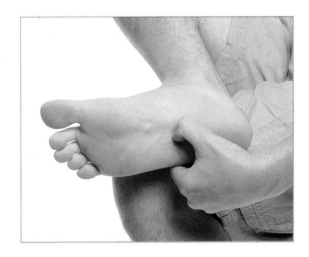

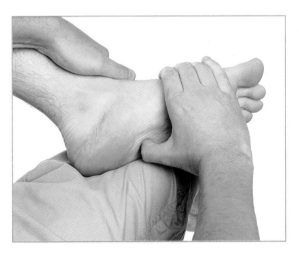

4 *Next, thumb-walk down the outside edge of your foot using your right thumb.*

5 *Finish by using your right thumb to thumb-walk across the heel to the inside of the foot again. Repeat the entire sequence three times.*

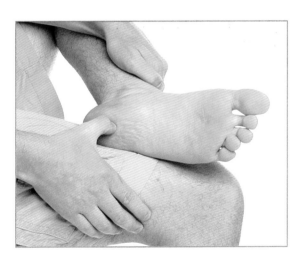

Energy-boosters

If fatigue has suddenly become a problem for you, you need to check with your doctor to ensure there is no underlying serious condition. For many people a daily energy slump is an annoying problem, rather than a true illness. Still, afternoon fatigue can interfere with your work and make life in general less enjoyable. Eating a well-balanced diet (which emphasizes high-quality protein) and getting regular cardiovascular exercise can help – as can these self-massage techniques. Just make sure that you use them before you get too tired.

Acupressure self-help

AIMS
to improve kidney and adrenal energy

FREQUENCY
at the onset of fatigue

CONTRAINDICATIONS
none known

CROSS-REFERENCE
Arthritis p. 28, Indigestion p. 50, Knee pain p. 54

ALSO BENEFICIAL FOR
BL 23 – dizziness, irritability, weakness
ST 36 – general well-being, weakness, pain below the navel

The acupoint Bladder 23 is known as the *Gate of Vitality*, and massaging this point can help to improve energy and concentration. Massaging Stomach 36, or *Three Mile Point*, is also known to improve energy levels.

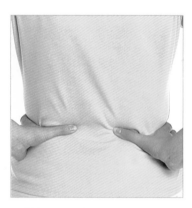

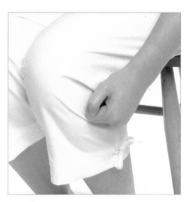

1 Wrap your hands around your waist and slide your thumbs towards each other. Feel for the band of muscle that runs along the spine on each side, then slide your thumbs up a little so that they are just below your ribs. This is the Gate of Vitality. Lean back into your thumbs and massage these areas in small circles. Continue for one minute.

2 Next, place your knuckles on Stomach 36, just below the kneecap on the outside of your shinbone on each leg. Rub this area briskly up and down for about one minute.

Reflexology quick fix

AIMS
to improve kidney and adrenal energy

FREQUENCY
as needed

CONTRAINDICATIONS
none known

CROSS-REFERENCE
Circulation issues p. 32

ALSO BENEFICIAL FOR
kidney complaints

Use the technique of rotating on a point (*see page 21*) on the adrenal-gland reflex zone, as shown below.

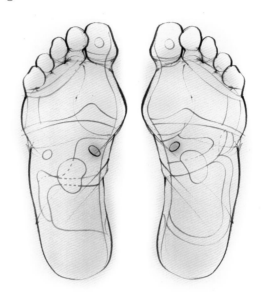

Self-massage quick fix

AIMS
to improve energy levels

FREQUENCY
at the onset of fatigue

CONTRAINDICATIONS
none known

CROSS-REFERENCE
Low backache p. 56

ALSO BENEFICIAL FOR
low backache

When your symptoms are not active, daily self-massage to the area can be very helpful in reducing pain and inflammation. It is important to emphasize range of motion techniques (moving the finger or hand in many different directions), which can help to break down restrictions in the joints.

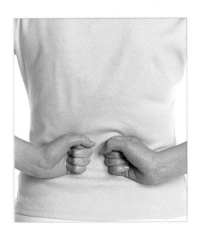

Make a fist and place your knuckles just under the ribs of your lower back. Rub vigorously for at least one minute.

Eye strain

Eye strain is especially common in computer users and others who do close work, such as sewing or knitting, and is exacerbated by poor lighting, glare from the computer or television, and not taking sufficient breaks. If you suffer from eye strain while you are working, make sure that you take a break every 15–30 minutes by looking away from your work and focusing on a distant object (at least 6 m/20 ft away) for 20 seconds. Here are some self-massage techniques that can help.

Acupressure self-help

AIMS
to relieve eye strain

FREQUENCY
several times a day

CONTRAINDICATIONS
none known

CROSS-REFERENCE
Computer strain p. 34, Hangovers p. 44, Mental clarity p. 62

ALSO BENEFICIAL FOR
ST 2 and 3 – sinus conditions, facial pain, headaches, dry eyes, head congestion
L 3 – headaches, hangovers, dizziness, allergies, foot cramps

This sequence, which can bring more energy (chi) to the eye area, will supplement breaks of focusing away from the work you are doing. If your work involves using your eyes intensely, use this self-treatment several times throughout the day.

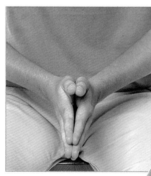

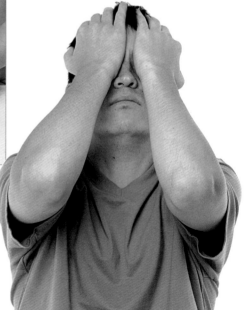

Begin by rubbing your hands together briskly until they are warm. Place your warm hands over your closed eyes and take two deep breaths. Repeat.

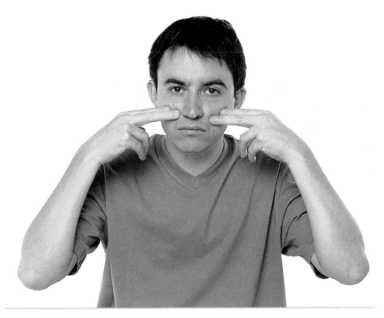

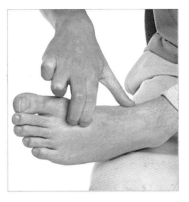

3 Place your right foot on your left thigh. Use your left index and middle fingers to massage Liver 3, located where the bones of the big and second toes meet, for one to two minutes (see above). You will feel a "zingy" or nervy sensation when you find the point. Repeat on your left foot.

2 Place your index and middle fingers respectively on Stomach 2, located at the centre of the cheekbone, and Stomach 3, located at the bottom of the cheekbone (both in line with the pupil). Massage this area in tiny circles for one to two minutes.

Reflexology self-help

AIMS
to relieve eye strain

FREQUENCY
as needed

CONTRAINDICATIONS
none known

ALSO BENEFICIAL FOR
headaches related to eye strain

This is a simple technique that can help ease eye strain. Use it while you are taking a break from your work or relaxing after work.

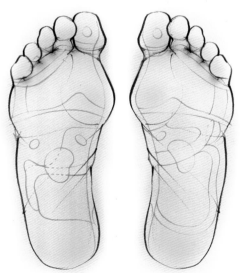

1 Locate the reflex area of the eyes on the foot, as shown here (see right). Rotate on the point and pinch (see pages 20–21) this area for about five minutes on each side.

Hangovers

Self-massage can help alleviate the symptoms of an occasional bout of over-indulgence, including headache, nausea and mental fuzziness. Because alcohol is a diuretic, it forces fluids out of the body and causes a loss of potassium. Eating a banana can help balance potassium loss and stabilize blood-sugar levels, and since bananas have an antacid effect, they can also help with nausea. Obviously drinking a lot of water the morning after can help address the dehydration brought on by a binge. Here are some massage techniques to try.

Indian head massage self-help

AIMS
to relieve headaches

FREQUENCY
several times the morning after a binge

CONTRAINDICATIONS
none known

CROSS-REFERENCE
Eye strain p. 42, Headaches p. 46

ALSO BENEFICIAL FOR
stimulating circulation, encouraging lymph flow, releasing toxins

You may want to try this self-massage while you are using a cold pack on your forehead.

1 *Lie down on the floor or a bed, or recline in a chair. With your fingertips, use circular friction to massage the muscles directly under the base of the skull. Start with your hands close to each other, just outside the spine, and work your way around to the ears. Continue for one to three minutes.*

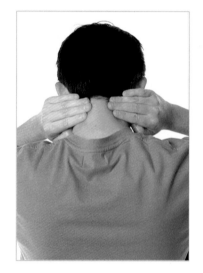

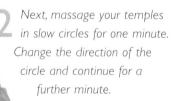

2 *Next, massage your temples in slow circles for one minute. Change the direction of the circle and continue for a further minute.*

Hydrotherapy quick fix

AIMS
to relieve headaches

FREQUENCY
several times the morning after a binge

CONTRAINDICATIONS
none known

CROSS-REFERENCE
Headaches p. 46

ALSO BENEFICIAL FOR
headaches from overeating or eating the wrong foods

The tried-and-trusted cold pack on the forehead is an excellent treatment for a hangover. Cold helps to shrink the blood vessels and can ameliorate a throbbing headache.

Use an ice pack wrapped in a towel. If you don't have an ice pack, place some ice cubes in a plastic bag, and wrap the bag in a towel. Apply this for about 10 minutes. Take a break, then prepare a fresh pack if necessary.

Acupressure quick fix

AIMS
to relieve headaches and nausea

FREQUENCY
three to five minutes on each point

CONTRAINDICATIONS
none known

ALSO BENEFICIAL FOR
L 3 – releasing toxins, soothing the eyes, clearing the mind
P 6 – insomnia, indigestion

Liver 3 is an excellent detox point. Pericardium 6 is famous for relieving nausea. Together these two acupoints may help you recover more quickly.

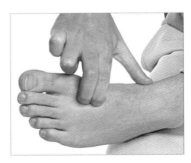

1 *Press Liver 3, located where the first and second toe bones meet on the top of the foot, on both feet for about one minute. You can also try massaging this point in small circles.*

2 *Press Pericardium 6, located on the inner arm, two-and-a-half finger widths above the wrist crease between the tendons, on the right arm for about one minute. You may prefer to massage this point in small circles. Repeat on the left arm.*

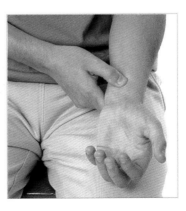

Headaches

If you suffer from mild, occasional headaches, you may be able to find relief with a few simple self-massage techniques. If you have frequent headaches or recurrent migraines, it is essential to get a diagnosis from a doctor and seek appropriate treatment. Here are some massage techniques that you can try for minor headaches.

Self-massage help for tension headaches

AIMS
to relieve the pain of a tension headache

FREQUENCY
repeat after one hour, if the first treatment does not resolve the headache or if the headache recurs

CONTRAINDICATIONS
none known

CROSS-REFERENCE
Neck and shoulder tension p. 66

ALSO BENEFICIAL FOR
stiff neck, tight shoulders

Tension headaches are often caused by muscle tightness in the neck and shoulders – this kind of headache will feel tight or squeezing. The good news is that tension headaches respond exceptionally well to self-massage.

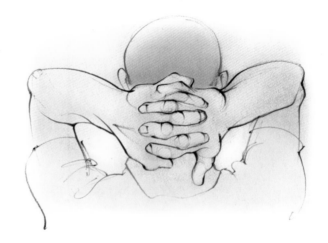

1 *Lie on the floor or sit in a chair and clasp your hands behind your neck. Squeeze and slide your palms towards each other. Repeat this action, starting from just under your skull and working your way down towards your shoulders. Continue for one minute.*

2 *Use your fingertips to massage the neck muscles on either side of the spine, using small, circular motions, from the base of the skull down to the shoulders. Massage for one to two minutes.*

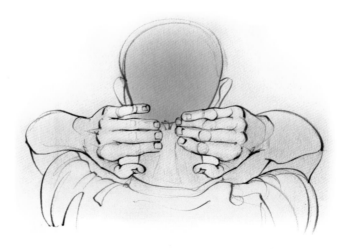

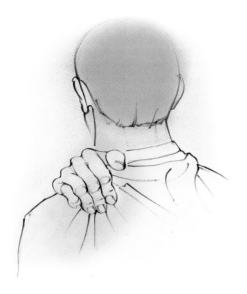

3 *Place your right hand on the thick band of muscle between the neck and shoulder on the left side. Cup the right elbow with the left hand for support. Squeeze and massage this area for at least one minute. Switch sides and repeat.*

Reflexology self-help for tension headaches

AIMS
to relieve the pain of a tension headache

FREQUENCY
repeat every 1–2 hours, as needed

CROSS-REFERENCE
Toothache p. 82

CONTRAINDICATIONS
none known

ALSO BENEFICIAL FOR
toothaches, sore throat, common cold

This treatment uses the reflex points associated with the spine and brain to help relieve the headache.

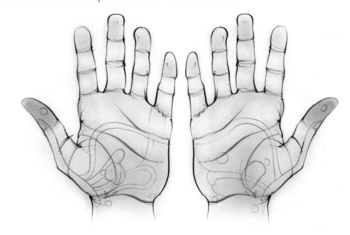

1 *Use your right thumb and index finger to pinch the tip of your left thumb (see right). Apply firm pressure and hold for five seconds. Repeat 10 times. Repeat the entire sequence on your right hand.*

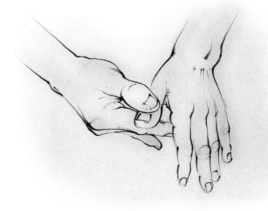

Acupressure self-help for sinus headaches

AIMS
to relieve the pain of a sinus headache

FREQUENCY
as needed

CONTRAINDICATIONS
none known

CROSS-REFERENCE
Eye strain p. 42, Toothache p. 82

ALSO BENEFICIAL FOR
blurry vision, eye strain, allergies, nasal congestion, facial swelling, toothache

This type of headache, which manifests in the forehead or around the eyes and cheeks, often responds extremely well to acupressure. You will be surprised at how quickly you feel the pressure being relieved by this treatment. If the sinus pressure returns after some time, simply repeat the sequence of points. Make sure you consult your physician if sinus conditions are a chronic problem for you.

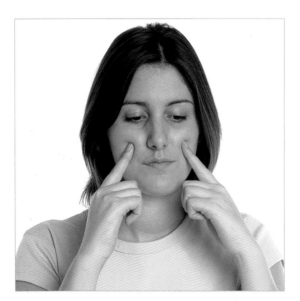

Using your index fingers, find Stomach 3, located at the bottom of the cheekbone below the eye on both sides. Massage these points gently in circles for one minute.

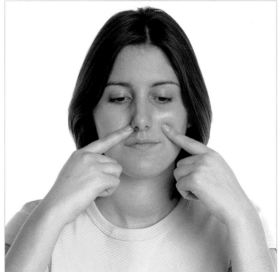

Determine which point is more tender, then continue to hold Stomach 3 on that side, while moving your other hand to Large Intestine 20, located just to the side of the nostril, on the other side. Massage both points in small circles for one minute.

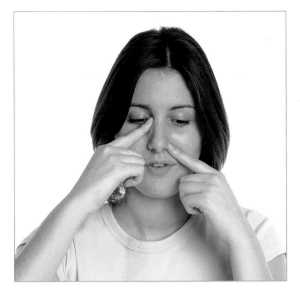

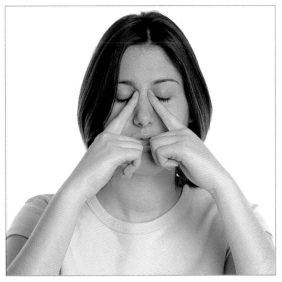

3 *Move the finger that is on Large Intestine 20 to Bladder 2, located on the inner corner of the eye, and hold. Move the finger that is still on Stomach 3 to Large Intestine 20 on the same side and massage in small circles for one minute.*

4 *Finish by holding Bladder 2 on both sides for a further minute. Rest and take several deep breaths.*

Acupressure self-help for digestive headaches

AIMS
to relieve a headache cause by digestive disturbances

FREQUENCY
several times a day

CONTRAINDICATIONS
pregnancy

CROSS-REFERENCE
Arthritis p. 28, Constipation p. 36, Joint mobility p. 52, Toothache p. 82

ALSO BENEFICIAL FOR
diarrhoea, constipation, rashes, tooth pain, facial tension

Some headaches are caused by digestive disturbances, such as overeating or constipation. One of the most well-known acupoints, Large Intestine 4, can help stimulate the digestive system to enable the body to get rid of the toxins that are causing the headache. You can use this treatment several times a day, until the headache eases.

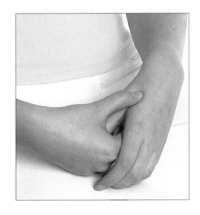

I *Place your right thumb on Large Intestine 4 on the left hand. Slide your right thumb down into the webbing between the fingers and press in towards of the index finger until you find a slightly nervy area.*
Massage this point in small circles for one to two minutes.

49

Indigestion

Indigestion is a catch-all term for things going wrong in the stomach and other parts of the digestive system – including heartburn, excessive burping and gas, and feelings of bloating and heaviness. These sensations may be accompanied by constipation or diarrhoea, nausea, vomiting, and/or a general feeling of weakness and fatigue. Indigestion can be caused by poor eating habits, such as eating too fast or too much, or eating excessively greasy food. Stress and anxiety, smoking and drinking alcohol also seem to aggravate (if not cause) indigestion. Allergies, lactose intolerance and lack of exercise may contribute to the problem.

Reflexology self-help

AIMS
to relieve heartburn

FREQUENCY
every hour until symptoms resolve, or once a day for improving symptoms in general

CONTRAINDICATIONS
none known

CROSS-REFERENCE
Constipation p. 36

ALSO BENEFICIAL FOR
diarrhoea, constipation, gas

It is important to understand which kind of indigestion you are experiencing and to treat it accordingly. Chronic indigestion can lead to other more serious health conditions, such as peptic ulcers, an inflamed oesophagus or gallstones. If you have chronic digestive problems, consult your doctor. Self-massage can complement other therapies, and here are some techniques for dealing with occasional indigestion.

When the lower sphincter of the oesophagus goes into spasms or is weak, gastric juice can easily splash up into the oesophagus and cause heartburn. Massaging this reflex zone can help diminish the severity of frequent heartburn.

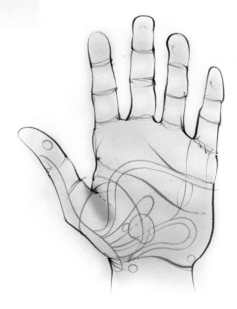

Use the technique of pinching and rotating on a point (see pages 20–21) on the reflex zone of the left hand, as shown here (left). Continue for two to three minutes.

Acupressure self-help

AIMS
to relieve indigestion

FREQUENCY
at the onset of symptoms, or twice a day for prevention

CONTRAINDICATIONS
none known

ALSO BENEFICIAL FOR
stomach pain, abdominal distension, diarrhoea, vomiting

This acupressure massage is helpful in relieving the symptoms of indigestion and strengthening the digestive system.

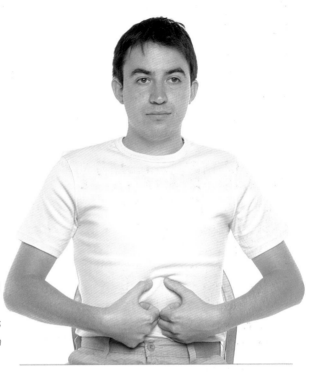

1 *Recline slightly in a chair. Place the thumbs of both hands on Conception Vessel 12, halfway between the bottom tip of the breastbone and the navel. Press in and slightly up. Massage gently with circular friction for up to two minutes.*

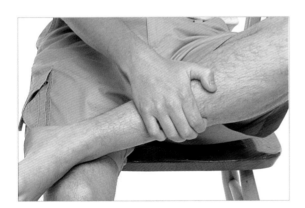

2 *Next, cross your left ankle over your right thigh. Use the fingertips of your right hand to stroke down the outside of your left shinbone, from just under the knee to the top of the foot. Continue stroking for two minutes.*

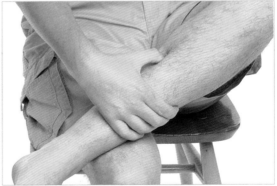

3 *Use your thumb to stroke upwards on your lower leg, just inside the shinbone, for two minutes. Repeat on the right leg.*

Joint mobility

Injuries, flu, cold weather, arthritis, overuse of the feet or hands and excessive acidity in the diet can all cause joint stiffness. In Chinese medicine, the joints are considered important places in the body, where the chi or energy gathers; many of the major acupoints are located in the wrists and ankles. Painful joints generally benefit from mild stretching (as long as there is no acute inflammation) and gentle massage. Daily massage to the wrists and ankles can help promote the flow of chi throughout the whole body. Here are some self-massage techniques to try.

Self-massage help

AIMS
to ease sore and aching joints in the hands

FREQUENCY
five-minute massage once or twice a day

CONTRAINDICATIONS
do not massage inflamed joints directly

CROSS-REFERENCE
Arthritis p. 28, Computer strain p. 34

ALSO BENEFICIAL FOR
carpal tunnel syndrome

A liniment such as Tiger Balm (or any camphor-based over-the-counter product) can make this massage more soothing. This sequence is designed for the wrist, but you can easily transfer it to the ankle.

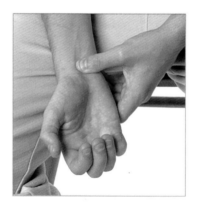

I *If you are using a liniment, begin by rubbing a generous amount into both the front and back of your wrist. If not, go straight to step 2.*

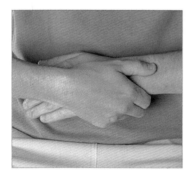

2 *Carefully massage the entire wrist joint. Start on the inside of your wrist and make small circles with your thumb all along the wrist crease. Continue for at least one minute. Next, make small circles in the area around the wrist crease. Continue for at least one minute.*

3 *Turn your hand over, hold the little-finger side of your hand with your fingers, and continue to use small circles with your thumb to massage the other side of your wrist. Continue for at least one minute.*

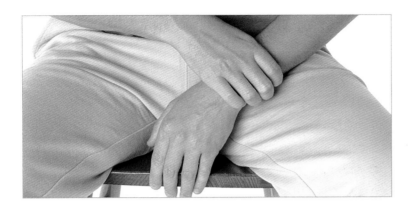

4 Turn your hand over again and grasp the wrist firmly with the fingers of the other hand. Squeeze gently several times. This action creates more space in the carpal tunnel. Finish with a hand massage (see page 28). Repeat steps 1–5 on the other side.

Trigger-point self-help

AIMS
to ease sore and aching ankles and feet

FREQUENCY
several times a day until the pain lessens

CONTRAINDICATIONS
limited mobility in the hips

CROSS-REFERENCE
Tired feet p. 80

Releasing this trigger point on your shin may help painful ankles and feet.

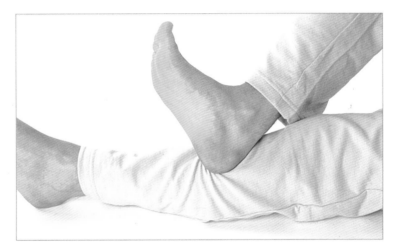

1 Sit either in a chair or on the floor. The first step in this massage is to find the trigger point. It is located on the outside of your shinbone, about one-third of the way down from the knee. Locating this point can be tricky because the muscles are usually very thick here. Lift your toes and you will feel a muscle on the outside of the shinbone pop out. Keeping your fingers on that muscle, relax your toes and then move your fingers down your shin about one-third of the way, feeling around for a tight or tender area.

2 Now place the heel of your opposite foot over this general area. Use the heel to rub the area strongly. Continue for one to two minutes. Repeat on the other leg. Finish your treatment with a soothing foot massage (see page 14).

Knee pain

Knee pain can be caused by arthritis, tendonitis, bursitis, damaged ligaments or cartilage, or very tight quadriceps muscles. It is important to understand the nature of chronic knee pain in order to treat it properly. If you have occasional knee pain, some of these self-massage techniques can be very helpful. If you have chronic knee pain, using one or more of the techniques daily will greatly complement any other treatment that you are receiving.

Trigger-point self-help

AIMS
to relieve knee pain, especially when accompanied by tight thigh muscles

FREQUENCY
daily

CONTRAINDICATIONS
none known

ALSO BENEFICIAL FOR
stiff thighs

Knee pain is often the result of thick knots in the quadriceps muscle, caused by over-exercise or over-exertion. If you have knee pain under the kneecap, try the first technique.

If the pain in your knee is a little above the knee joint, you may want to try this second trigger point.

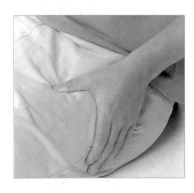

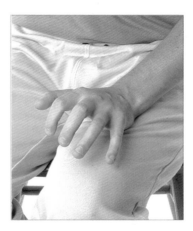

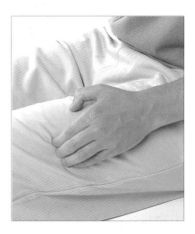

1 *Place your thumb on the top of the thigh, just below the groin. Move your thumb around until you find a tight or "knotty" area. Massage this area in small circles with both thumbs, or use the outside of your wrist. Continue for three to five minutes.*

2 *Place your thumb on the centre top of the thigh, equidistant from the groin and the top of the knee. Move your thumb around until you find a tight or "knotty" area. It should feel tender or even painful. Massage this area in small circles with the thumbs, or use the outside of the heel of your hand for three to five minutes.*

3 *Next, feel the outside of your thigh and notice if this area is also tight. If it is, take a few minutes to massage it with the fingertips of both hands, working from the upper thigh towards the knee joint.*

Acupressure self-help

AIMS
to relieve knee pain (especially useful for arthritis)

FREQUENCY
two to three times a day

CONTRAINDICATIONS
if you have had recent knee surgery, consult your doctor

CROSS-REFERENCE
Arthritis p. 28, Constipation p. 36, Energy-boosters p. 40

ALSO BENEFICIAL FOR
constipation, stomach problems, fatigue

You will find this massage will be especially beneficial if you practise it daily.

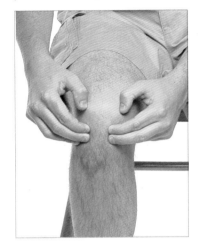
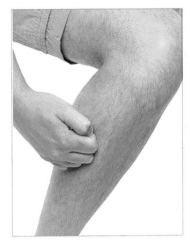

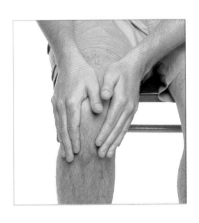

1 Begin by briskly rubbing the knee between both palms. Massage the muscles around the knee (left). Continue for about two minutes.

2 Find acupoint "Xiyan" (it is an "extra" point and does not have a number), located just below the kneecap on either side

of the tendon. Massage both sides of the tendon with the index and middle fingers of both hands for about one minute (above, left).

3 Next, use your knuckles to rub Stomach 36, located about four finger widths below the kneecap on the outside of the shinbone, for about one minute.

Reflexology quick fix

AIMS
to relieve knee pain

FREQUENCY
once a day, or more

CONTRAINDICATIONS
none known

ALSO BENEFICIAL FOR
hip and leg pain

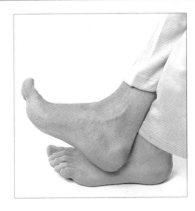

1 Remove your shoes. Use the heel of the right foot to press the outside of the left foot, as shown here. Continue for about two minutes. Repeat on the other side.

2 Alternatively, place the left foot on top of the right thigh and stimulate the top of your left foot with your fingers.

Low backache

At one time or another about 90 per cent of the population will experience lower back pain. A variety of situations can create low backache, including poor posture, prolapsed intervertebral discs, strained muscles or ligaments, inflammation of the pelvic joints, chronic constipation and pre-menstrual tension. Backache is sometimes combined with sciatica, a pain that travels down the leg. Back pain often responds well to professional massage, chiropractic care and/or physical therapy. The following self-massage techniques can complement professional treatment.

Self-massage help

AIMS
to relieve backache

FREQUENCY
several times a day

CONTRAINDICATIONS
none known

CROSS-REFERENCE
Energy-boosters p. 40, Do-in self-massage p. 86

ALSO BENEFICIAL FOR
sciatica, paralysis of the lower extremities

This is a simple massage that you can do at work or home, sitting in a firm chair.

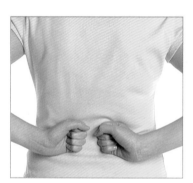

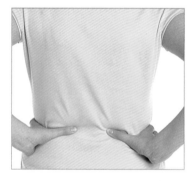

1 *Make fists and lean forward slightly. Place the knuckles on either side of your spine and rub briskly up and down and from side to side. Continue for about one minute.*

2 *Next, place your hands on your waist with the thumbs pointing backwards and press into the tight lower back muscles and the sacrum. Lean back into your thumbs. Move your thumbs to a new spot and then lean back again. Use circular massage for a few seconds before moving your thumbs to another spot. Continue pressing into your back like this for one or two minutes.*

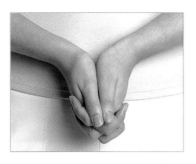 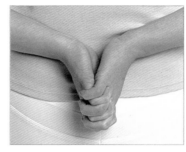

3 *Now clasp your hands behind your back with the thumbs straight and pressed against each other. Tap or pound the thumb side of your hand against your sacrum. Continue for about one minute.*

Lower back pain can also be the result of very tight hamstring muscles (the muscles in the back of your thigh). Many people hold stress in their hamstrings the way others hold it in their neck and shoulders. Stretching and massaging your hamstrings can greatly benefit your lower back.

1 *Use the backs of your hands to strongly tap the back of your thighs. It may feel good to use a lot of pressure. Tap for about one minute.*

2 *Next, knead the back of your thigh with both hands. Continue for about one minute. Repeat steps 1 and 2 on your other leg.*

3 *When you've finished massaging the backs of your legs, stretch them both out in front of you. Place your hands on your shins or your ankles and gently lean forward. If you feel the stretch in your lower back, try flexing your feet. You should mainly feel the stretch in the backs of your legs.*

Acupressure self-help

AIMS
to relieve backache

FREQUENCY
several times a day

CONTRAINDICATIONS
none known

CROSS-REFERENCE
Menstrual discomfort p. 60

ALSO BENEFICIAL FOR
sciatica, paralysis of the lower extremities

Some of the best acupoints for treating lower backache are in the leg and ankle. These points are easy to access and can help relieve minor symptoms.

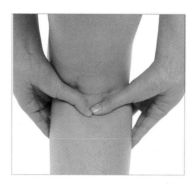 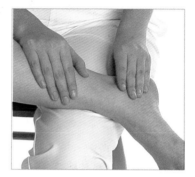

1 *Find Bladder 40 on your right leg, located in the centre of the back of the knee (see top left). It may feel very tight. Use your thumbs to gently massage this point for one to two minutes.*

2 *Next, place your right foot on your left thigh and find Bladder 60, located between the Achilles tendon and the outer ankle bone. Massage for one to two minutes with your thumb. Repeat on the left leg.*

Reflexology self-help

AIMS
to relieve backache

FREQUENCY
several times a day

CONTRAINDICATIONS
none known

CROSS-REFERENCE
Menstrual discomfort p. 60

ALSO BENEFICIAL FOR
sciatica, paralysis of the lower extremities

The inside of the foot, from the heel to the big toe, holds many reflex points for the spine. Massaging this whole area can benefit the lower back. If your hips or back are too stiff to place your foot on top of your opposite thigh, try the reflex points on your hands, as shown on page 59.

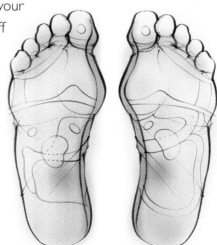

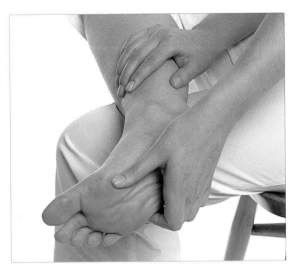

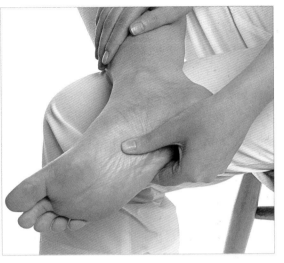

| Grasp the inside of the right foot with both hands. Twist and wring the inside of the foot. Then use your left thumb to thumb-walk (see page 21) up the inside of the arch, from heel to toe. Continue for one to two minutes.

2 Next, use your left thumb to thumb-walk up the lower half of your foot arch. Continue for one to two minutes. Repeat on the left foot.

Hand reflexology quick fix

AIMS
to relieve backache

FREQUENCY
several times a day

CONTRAINDICATIONS
none known

ALSO BENEFICIAL FOR
sciatica

If your hips or back are too stiff to place your foot on top of your opposite thigh to massage your feet, try the reflex points in your hands, as shown below.

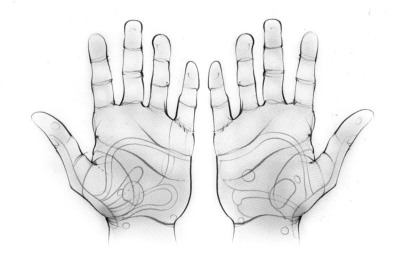

| Thumb-walk (see page 21) over the reflex area, as shown here. Continue for about two minutes. Repeat several times a day.

Menstrual discomfort

Discomfort before, during or after menstruation can be caused by a variety of factors, including tight lower back muscles and/or pelvic muscles, hormonal imbalances, lack of exercise, anaemia and constipation. It is important to consult your doctor to try to understand the underlying causes of your specific menstruation-related symptoms and get appropriate treatment. These simple self-massage techniques may help.

Self-massage help

AIMS
to relieve the lower back pain and pelvic tension that cause menstrual discomfort

FREQUENCY
once or twice a day

CONTRAINDICATIONS
none known

CROSS-REFERENCE
Low backache p. 56

ALSO BENEFICIAL FOR
low backache, sciatica

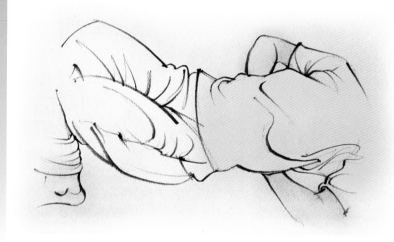

1 Lie down on your back on a carpeted floor or padded surface. Raise your knees and bring your feet up flat on the floor. Lift your hips and slide your fists under your lower back, with the knuckles facing up, on either side of the spine. Gently rock your hips from side to side, allowing the back muscles to be massaged. (You can also try this technique with tennis balls. Put two in a sock, tie the top and place under your back. Rock your hips from side to side.)

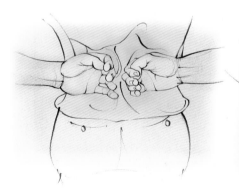

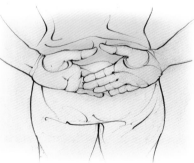

2 Next, lift your hips and flatten your palms to the floor. Slide your hands down to your sacrum (lower back). Lower your hips onto your hands. Continue to rock from side to side and in circles, massaging the sacrum.

Acupressure self-help

AIMS
to relieve menstrual discomfort

FREQUENCY
two to three times a day, beginning one week before the onset of your period

CONTRAINDICATIONS
do not use this acupoint to relieve any discomfort during the last two months of pregnancy because it can initiate labour

CROSS-REFERENCE
Low backache p. 56

ALSO BENEFICIAL FOR
water retention, genital pain, stomach discomfort

This acupoint is well known for its beneficial effects on all sorts of menstrual discomfort. Use it several times a day in the week leading up to menstruation, then during the first few days of your period when you have discomfort.

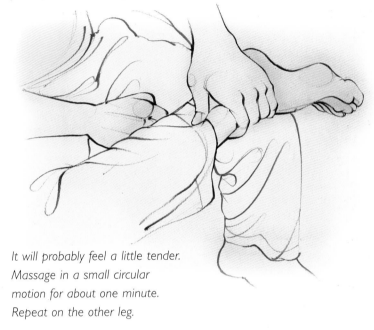

Place your right foot on top of your left thigh and find Spleen 6, located four finger widths above the top of the inner ankle bone, just on the inside of the shinbone.

It will probably feel a little tender. Massage in a small circular motion for about one minute. Repeat on the other leg.

Hand reflexology quick fix

AIMS
to relieve menstrual discomfort

FREQUENCY
several times a day

CONTRAINDICATIONS
none known

ALSO BENEFICIAL FOR
the brain and the pituitary gland

This easy technique can be used at any time, anywhere.

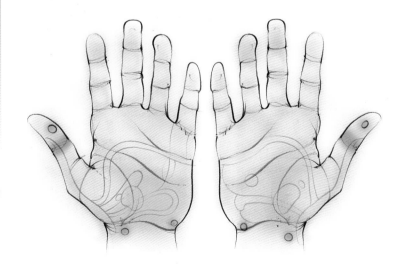

Use the pinching technique (see page 21) on the first knuckle of each thumb, as shown here (right). Stimulate the crease of this knuckle for about one minute.

Mental clarity

If the neck is stiff and tight, blood flow to the brain is constricted and this can result in mental fatigue. Unfortunately, many of us assume a poor posture when we are doing concentrated mental work. Sitting slumped or without proper support of the lower back for long hours at a computer can contribute to tension in the neck, shoulders and back of the head. Massaging your shoulders and correcting postural misalignments may be very helpful in staving off mental fatigue and fogginess. Try these self-help techniques.

Self-massage help

AIMS
to improve mental clarity

FREQUENCY
at least twice a day, during breaks from work

CONTRAINDICATIONS
for serious neck injury, such as whiplash, check first with your doctor

CROSS-REFERENCE
Headaches p. 46, Neck and shoulder tension p. 66

ALSO BENEFICIAL FOR
stiff neck and shoulders, tension headaches

AROMATHERAPY TIP
mix a few drops of grapefruit, peppermint or rosemary essential oil with a carrier oil on your hands and rub them together before beginning this massage. These essential oils are well known for their ability to improve mental clarity.

This simple exercise takes just five minutes and provides a great deal of relief.

1 *Lie on the floor or sit in a chair. With your fingertips, massage your temples in small, slow circles. Continue for about one minute. Change the direction of your circles and continue massaging for another minute.*

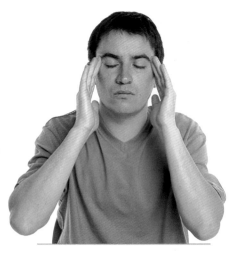

2 *Next, clasp your hands behind your neck. Squeeze and slide your palms towards each other. Repeat this action, starting from just under your skull and working your way down towards your shoulders. Continue for about one minute.*

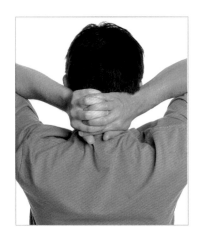

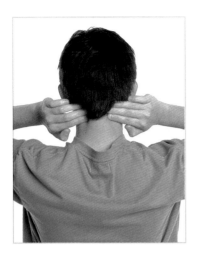

3 Now use your fingertips to massage the neck muscles on either side of the spine, using circular friction, from the base of the skull down to the shoulders. Massage for one to two minutes.

4 Place your right hand on your left shoulder. Support your right elbow with the left hand. Knead and use circular friction on this area for two minutes. Pay special attention to any knots.

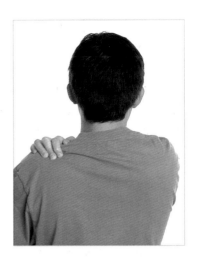

Acupressure quick fix

AIMS
to improve mental clarity

FREQUENCY
several times a day

CONTRAINDICATIONS
none known

CROSS-REFERENCE
Eye strain p. 42, Headaches p. 46

ALSO BENEFICIAL FOR
tension headaches, poor memory, pain that inhibits the ability to concentrate, dizziness, cold symptoms including sinus congestion, swollen eyes

The healing property of this acupoint is suggested in its name The *Gates of Consciousness*. This point has a variety of uses, many of which are directly related to brain function.

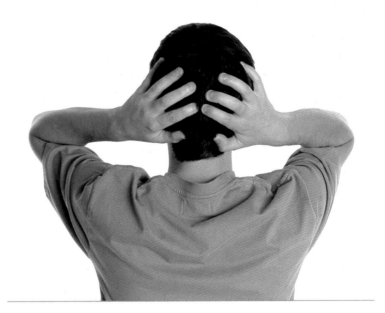

1 Sit in a straight-backed chair. Place your thumbs behind the ears and just under your skull on each side. Relax your head back into your hands and against the chair back. Now slide your thumbs towards the back of your head.

Stop just before you come to the thick muscle band – this is the acupoint. Your thumbs will be about 5–7.5 cm/2–3 in apart. Massage for about one minute. You can also do this massage lying on your back.

Reflexology quick fix

AIMS
to improve mental clarity

FREQUENCY
several times a day

CONTRAINDICATIONS
none known

CROSS-REFERENCE
Headaches p. 46

ALSO BENEFICIAL FOR
dizziness, fainting, fever

Stimulating the brain reflex area can help dissipate mental fatigue. This is a great technique because you can do it in the middle of a business meeting, on an aeroplane, or anywhere else when you need a quick boost.

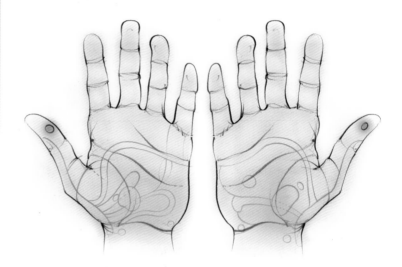

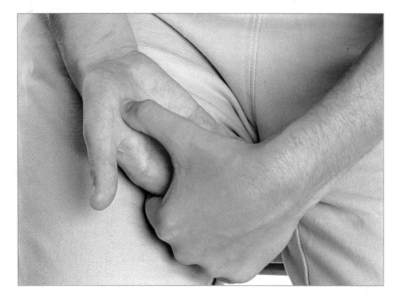

Use the technique of pinching and rotating on a point (see pages 20–21) in the centre of the pad of the thumb for about two minutes. Repeat on the other hand.

Muscle cramps

Muscles can cramp up as a result of overuse, which is why athletes are often plagued with this condition. Simply massaging the cramped muscle and stretching the area often works to relieve the cramp. Sometimes muscle cramps are related to mineral imbalances in the diet. If you suffer from frequent muscle cramps, see your doctor. Here are some self-massage techniques to help with occasional muscle cramps.

Acupressure self-help for muscle cramps

AIMS
to relieve muscle cramps

FREQUENCY
repeat whenever cramping occurs

CONTRAINDICATIONS
none known

ALSO BENEFICIAL FOR
headaches, allergies, arthritis, eye strain

The acupoint Liver 3 is recommended for muscle cramps in general, and specifically for foot cramps.

Place your right foot on your left thigh. Use your left index and middle fingers to massage the area where the bones of the big and second toes meet, for about one minute. You will feel a "zingy" or nervy sensation when you find the point. Repeat on your left foot.

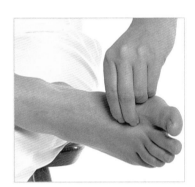

Acupressure self-help for leg cramps

AIMS
to relieve cramp in the calf muscle

FREQUENCY
repeat whenever cramping recurs

CONTRAINDICATIONS
none known

CROSS-REFERENCE
Low backache p. 56

ALSO BENEFICIAL FOR
lower back pain and sciatica

Massaging the acupoint Bladder 57 can help relieve a cramp in the calf muscle. Even if you only have cramp in one leg, it is good to massage the point on both sides of the body.

To find Bladder 57, slide your thumb straight down the middle of your calf muscle, until you come to the bottom of the muscle. This is the point. If your calf is in spasm, this will be very easy to feel. Use your thumb to massage this point until the spasm resolves. Repeat on your other calf.

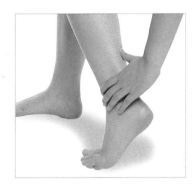

Neck and shoulder tension

For most people, neck and shoulder tension is an unfortunate symptom of modern life. During the 10 years I have worked as a massage therapist, almost all of my clients have complained, at one time or another (if not at every visit), of sore shoulders and/or a stiff neck. The cause can often be traced to everyday posture – including working at a desk, typing on a computer, slouching in front of the television and driving a car. In addition to bad posture, poor digestion can also be a factor. Two important meridians, the Gall Bladder and Small Intestine, run through the neck and shoulder area. Modifying your diet by cutting down on greasy foods and salt, and eating slowly and in a relaxed mood, can often help to eliminate some neck and shoulder tension.

Self-massage help

AIMS
to relieve neck and shoulder tension

This is a short treatment that you can easily do while sitting at your desk.

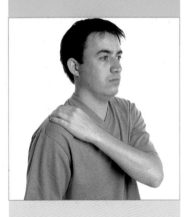

FREQUENCY
once or twice a day for chronic conditions, more often for acute

CONTRAINDICATIONS
none known

CROSS-REFERENCE
Headaches p. 46

ALSO BENEFICIAL FOR
tension headaches

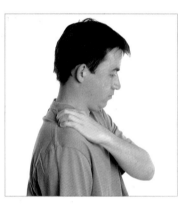

1 *Make a fist with your right hand, but keep the fist loose at the wrist. Support your right elbow with your left hand if necessary. Tilt your head slightly to the right and pound your fist (with as much strength as you like) into the hard muscle band that runs on top of your shoulder up into your neck. Continue for about one minute, then repeat on the other side.*

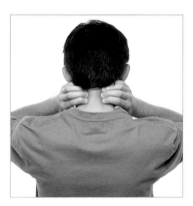

2 *Squeeze the same area on top of your shoulder with your right hand. Slide your hand from the shoulder up to the neck and squeeze the neck muscles for about one minute. Repeat on the other side.*

3 *Use your fingertips to massage the neck muscles on both sides of the spine, using small, circular motions, from the base of the skull down to the shoulders. Massage for one to two minutes.*

Reflexology quick fix

AIMS
to relieve neck and shoulder tension

FREQUENCY
several times a day

CONTRAINDICATIONS
none known

CROSS-REFERENCE
Stress p. 74

ALSO BENEFICIAL FOR
general overall tension, ulcers, whiplash, headache, fainting

This simple technique won't wear you out. If you are too tired or sore to give yourself a neck and shoulder massage, try the reflex zone in your hands.

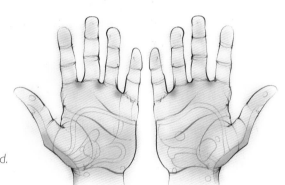

1 *Pinch the area between the fingers, then thumb walk down the edge of the thumb to the palm. Continue for about two minutes. Repeat on the other hand.*

Trigger-point self-help

AIMS
to relieve neck and shoulder tension

FREQUENCY
twice a day, or more often

CONTRAINDICATIONS
none known

CROSS-REFERENCE
Headaches p. 46

ALSO BENEFICIAL FOR
headache, jaw pain

Almost everyone will experience a tightness in the two trigger points of the trapezius at some time or another. These points can cause a lot of the tension on top of the shoulder, in the neck and between the shoulder blade and spine. Some simple self-massage will help to bring relief. Trigger-point therapy generally works best when you repeat it daily for a week or more.

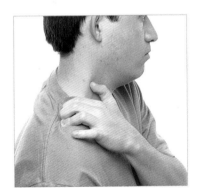

1 *Find the thick muscle roll on top of your opposite shoulder. Move your fingers around this area until you find the sorest spot – this is the trigger point.*

It is not very deep, and it might feel about as thick as a pencil under your fingers. Massage this point with the fingertips for about two minutes. Repeat on the other side.

2 *Next, lie on the floor with a tennis ball under your back, between your shoulder blade and your spine. Roll around your shoulder blade until you find the sorest area. Massage this area by rolling up and down, and back and forth for about two minutes. Repeat on the other side.*

Pregnancy discomfort

Self-massage can be helpful in addressing a variety of pregnancy-related discomforts, from nausea and heartburn to sore feet and back pain. It is always a great idea to get a professional massage or have your partner massage you when you are feeling the strain of pregnancy; however, these self-help techniques can also bring great relief.

Aromatherapy massage self-help

AIMS
to relieve sore feet, fatigue, general ill feeling and emotional sensitivity

FREQUENCY
once a day, generally in the evening

Choose an essential oil such as lavender, eucalyptus, orange or rose to mix with a few tablespoons of pure vegetable oil, such as sesame, almond or sunflower. Lavender essential oil is a good choice for its relaxing, pain-relieving qualities; you may want to try eucalyptus or orange if you feel as though you need a pick-me-up, or rose if you're feeling particularly blue.

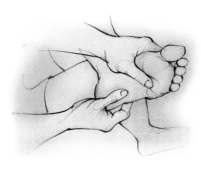 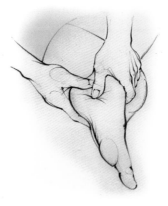 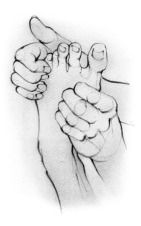

CONTRAINDICATIONS
be careful not to spend too much time on the little toe or just above the inner ankle bone next to the shinbone, as these are both points that can initiate labour avoid rose oil during the first four months of pregnancy

CROSS-REFERENCE
Tired feet p. 80

1 *After soaking your feet in hot water for a few minutes, dry them and sit in a comfortable chair. Spread a towel across your thigh and rest the opposite foot on the towel. Use about one teaspoon of your oil mixture and begin to work it into the sole of your foot with slow sweeping thumb strokes.*

2 *Pay special attention to the inside of your heel, below and to the side of the ankle bone. Make sure you massage each toe.*

3 *Massage the top of your foot with your fingers. Stroke between the bones. Continue for about five minutes on each foot. When you are finished, prop your feet up (making sure you keep them warm) and relax.*

Acupressure self-help

AIMS
to relieve nausea

FREQUENCY
can be used whenever nausea arises

CONTRAINDICATIONS
none known

CROSS-REFERENCE
Sinus congestion and pain p. 70

ALSO BENEFICIAL FOR
insomnia, palpitations, epilepsy, motion sickness

This acupoint is well known for its ability to control nausea and vomiting and can be used safely during all stages of pregnancy. It is also excellent for controlling motion sickness.

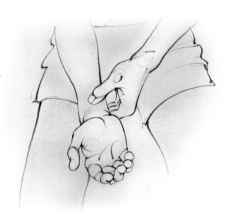

Find Pericardium 6, located two-and-a-half finger widths above the wrist crease, between the tendons in the centre of your forearm. Press the point deeply with your thumb and hold the pressure firmly for five to ten long, slow breaths. Repeat on the other side.
Continue on alternate sides until the nausea subsides.

Self-massage help for heartburn

AIMS
to quell heartburn

FREQUENCY
whenever the symptom arises; use preventively towards the end of pregnancy

CONTRAINDICATIONS
none known

CROSS-REFERENCE
Mental clarity p. 62, Stress p. 74

ALSO BENEFICIAL FOR
calming the mind

Perform this massage over your clothing. The technique works best in conjunction with other natural therapies such as taking a calcium supplement or digestive enzymes.

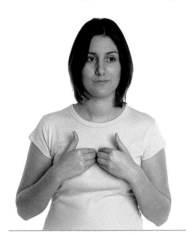

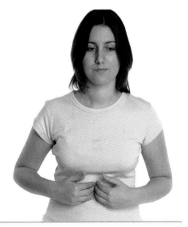

1 *Use your fingertips to stroke down the breastbone. Begin at the notch in your collar bone and slide your fingers down to your abdomen. Repeat for one minute.*

2 *Next, using the same stroking motion, slide your fingers straight down to the top of your abdomen. Use light pressure if you are in your last trimester.*

Sinus congestion and pain

Sinuses may become irritated by allergies, colds or flu. Both acute and chronic sinus problems can indicate a more serious condition that needs to be evaluated and treated by a doctor. Self-massage can be an excellent adjunct to other therapies.

Acupressure self-help

AIMS
to relieve sinus congestion and pain

FREQUENCY
several times a day

CONTRAINDICATIONS
none known

CROSS-REFERENCE
Eye strain p. 42, Neck and shoulder tension p. 66

ALSO BENEFICIAL FOR
ST 3 – eye irritation, sinus headaches, facial pain
BL 10 – headache, rigidity of the neck

These two acupoints can help clear up blocked sinuses and may be used at any time, anywhere.

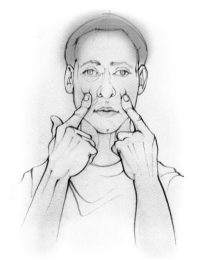

1 *Find Stomach 3 by placing both index fingers under your cheekbones and pressing up into the bone. Rub your fingers back and forth along the ridge of the bone until you feel a slight depression in it – this is the acupoint. It will probably be tender – more so on the side where you are feeling greater congestion.*

2 *Hold the point with firm, steady pressure on both sides and take 10 deep breaths.*

3 *Next, find Bladder 10 by placing your thumbs into the muscles on either side of the spine at the base of the skull. This acupoint is right on the muscle band. Tilt your head slightly forward and begin to massage the area, making slow, deep circles with your thumbs. Even if you are not exactly on the acupoint, massage of this area will feel good and will help relieve sinus congestion. Massage this point for about two minutes.*

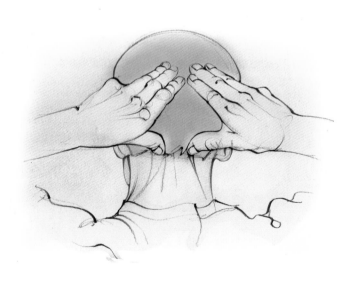

Reflexology self-help

AIMS
to relieve sinus congestion and pain

FREQUENCY
twice a day

CONTRAINDICATIONS
none known

ALSO BENEFICIAL FOR
facial pain

Massaging the reflex zones on both the hands and the feet can help soothe the sinuses. Remember, in general, the feet are a more effective treatment area, but if you are in a situation where you can't massage your feet easily, the hands are a great substitute.

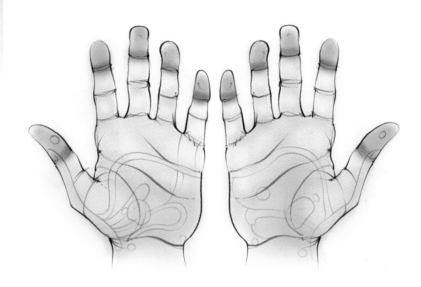

1 *Use the technique of pinching and rotating on a point (see pages 20–21) in the reflex zones on the hands, as shown here. Repeat on each digit for about one minute.*

2 *The sinus reflex zones in the feet are located in the corresponding places (right). Repeat the pinching and rotating technique on the feet.*

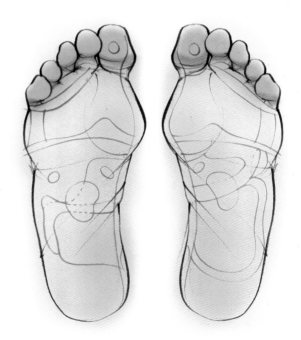

Sleeplessness

Just about everyone has trouble sleeping sometimes. The causes can range from drinking too much coffee during the day to anxiety and not getting enough exercise. Jetlag, the side-effects of medication and back pain can also cause occasional insomnia. If you are experiencing chronic insomnia, it is essential to see your doctor for appropriate treatment. If you have infrequent bouts of sleeplessness, self-massage can help you relax and get a good night's rest. The following techniques can help.

Acupressure self-help

AIMS
to relieve insomnia

FREQUENCY
as needed

CONTRAINDICATIONS
none known

CROSS-REFERENCE
Eye strain p. 42, Menstrual discomfort p. 62

ALSO BENEFICIAL FOR
BL 62 – eye strain, epileptic fits at night
KD 6 – irregular menstruation, prolapsed uterus

You can use this treatment in bed just before trying to get to sleep, or if you wake up in the middle of the night and cannot get back to sleep.

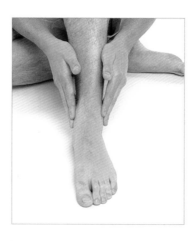

1 *Find Bladder 62, located on the outside of the ankle, about a thumb width directly beneath the bottom of the ankle bone. Kidney 6 is directly opposite Bladder 62, beneath the inside of the ankle bone.*

2 *Use the fingertips of both hands to massage these points in slow, circular strokes for about two minutes. Repeat on the other ankle.*

3 *If you are lying in bed and don't want to sit up, try using the heel of your opposite foot to massage the area beneath the inner ankle bone. Continue for about two minutes on each side and then relax. Repeat if necessary.*

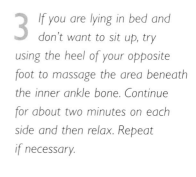

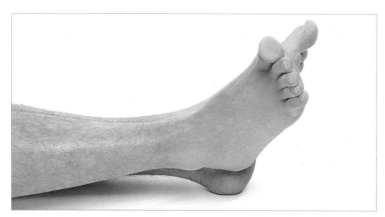

Reflexology self-help

AIMS
to relax the body and mind in order to fall asleep

FREQUENCY
repeat until you fall asleep

CONTRAINDICATIONS
none known

ALSO BENEFICIAL FOR
sinus problems, headaches, blood sugar problems

Use the pinching and rotating technique (see pages 20–21) on the reflex zones of the hands as shown here. Repeat on each digit for about one minute.

The reflex zones on both of the hands can be useful in easing insomnia – and you can treat yourself while lying down.

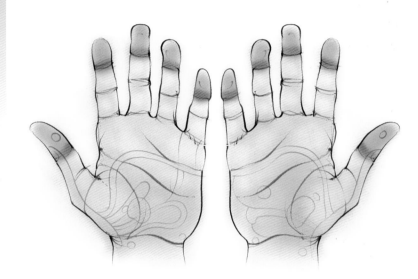

Meditation help

AIMS
to relieve insomnia

FREQUENCY
daily

CONTRAINDICATIONS
none known

ALSO BENEFICIAL FOR
general anxiety, tension

Try this simple meditation to help you get a restful night's sleep.
1. Lie comfortably, either on your back or your side.
2. Close your eyes and breathe deeply through your nose. Concentrate on the breath coming in through your nose and slowly leaving through your nose.
3. Now take your awareness to your feet. As you breathe in, tell yourself, "my feet are heavy." As you breathe out, tell yourself, "my feet are relaxed." Repeat this phrase with the breath three times. Feel a warm relaxing sensation spread through your feet.
4. Next, take your mind to your ankles. As you breathe in, tell yourself, "my ankles are heavy." As you breathe out, tell yourself, "my ankles are relaxed." Feel the warm relaxing sensation spread from your feet into your ankles. Repeat three times.
5. Continue this meditation with each part of your body. If you have not fallen asleep by the time you reach your head, begin the process again.

Stress

In today's fast-paced world it is hard to find anyone who doesn't experience occasional stress. One of the best things you can do for yourself when you are under stress is to take a break and get a massage. In fact, stress reduction is one of the most highly touted benefits of massage therapy. While it is great to receive a massage from a professional, self-massage can help too. Try one of the following techniques and see which works best for you.

Indian head-massage self-help

AIMS
to ease stress and tension

FREQUENCY
daily

CONTRAINDICATIONS
none known

CROSS-REFERENCE
Energy-boosters p. 40, Eye strain p. 42, Headaches p. 46

ALSO BENEFICIAL FOR
headaches, fatigue, tired eyes

Indian head massage has been used for centuries to help relieve stress and tension. Here is a simple routine that will take you less than five minutes.

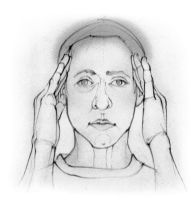

1 *Lie down or sit in a chair. Begin by using your fingertips to rub your temples in small, slow circles. Continue for about one minute.*

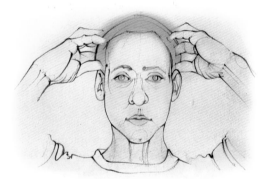

2 *Next "shampoo" your scalp. Begin just behind the temples and make small circles, rubbing towards the back of your head. Massage the whole scalp. Continue for at least one minute.*

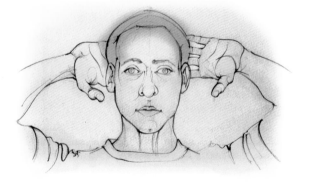

3 *Finish by "combing" your scalp with your fingertips, from the hairline, over the top and sides of the head and down the back of your neck to the shoulders. Repeat this stroke about 10 times.*

Reflexology quick fix

AIMS
to relieve stress

FREQUENCY
several times a day

CONTRAINDICATIONS
none known

CROSS-REFERENCE
Energy-boosters p. 40

ALSO BENEFICIAL FOR
fatigue

You can use this massage when you are under a lot of stress, but don't have time to take care of yourself with a longer self-massage treatment. The benefit of hand reflexology is that it can be performed without other people becoming aware of it, so the treatment can be done during a stressful meeting or while commuting.

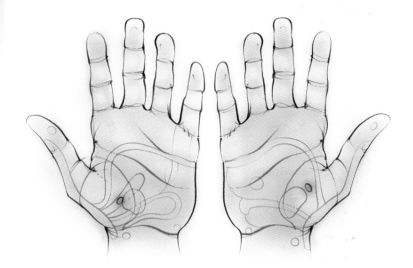

1 *Use the techniques of pinching or rotating on a point (see pages 20–21) on the reflex zone, as shown above Continue for up to five minutes on each hand.*

2 *Alternately, place a marble or a small, hard ball between your palms and squeeze them towards each other. Roll the ball around the inner part of your palm.*

Meditation help

AIMS
to relieve stress

FREQUENCY
twice a day or more

CONTRAINDICATIONS
none known

ALSO BENEFICIAL FOR
sleep issues, anxiety

Meditation is a tried and true remedy for stress. Because the point of meditation is to concentrate the mind, it can help divert your mind from the cause of your stress long enough to realize it is manageable. In the past few years, much research has been done to confirm that meditation helps reduce stress and promotes healing. Here is a short meditation to help you cope with stress.

1. Sit in a comfortable position – either cross-legged on the floor or in a chair.

2. Close your eyes and breathe slowly and deeply through your nose. Concentrate on the breath coming in and out through your nose. Count from down from ten to one. You can visualize the numbers in your head if it helps you to focus on breathing and ignore other thoughts.

3. When you get to one, repeat the count down again. You may want to repeat it a few more times before proceeding to the next step.

4. Take your awareness to the centre of your chest. Feel a gentle warmth and love in this part of your body. Over the next few breaths, allow that feeling of warmth and love to spread out from your heart until you feel your whole body gently radiating with it. If your mind wanders, allow your awareness to come back to the centre of the chest. Whenever a stressful thought arises, imagine wrapping it up in the warm, healing energy of your heart until you feel it dissolve there. Continue this meditation for at least 10 minutes and use it whenever you need to relieve stress.

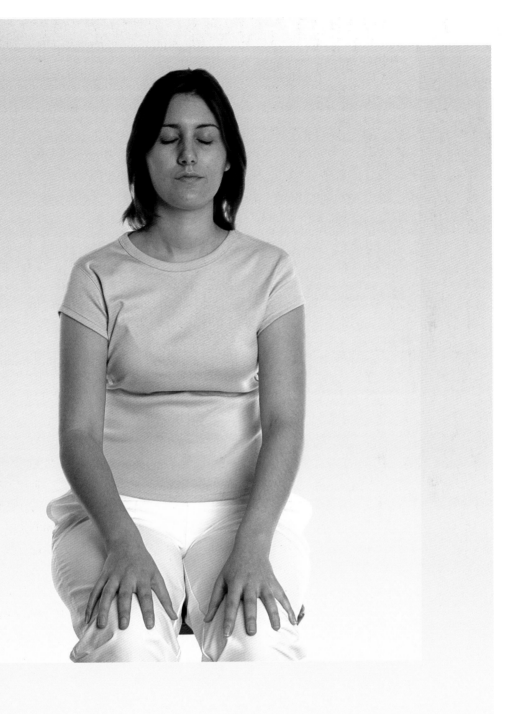

Swelling

Water retention and swelling (also known as oedema) can be an annoying nuisance or a serious problem. Swelling from kidney, liver or heart disease, diabetes, AIDS or other diseases is a condition which needs to be treated by a physician. In any case, it is generally not a good idea to give yourself a firm, deep massage over an area that is swollen. However, a specific kind of massage therapy, known as manual lymphatic drainage, is tremendously beneficial for it. This therapy is most effective when performed by a trained professional, although simple self-massage can bring relief from minor swelling.

Manual lymphatic drainage self-help

AIMS
to help reduce swelling

FREQUENCY
twice a day

CONTRAINDICATIONS
consult a doctor about your specific condition

CROSS-REFERENCE
Circulation issues p. 32, Knee pain p. 54, Pregnancy discomfort p. 68, Tired feet p. 80

Manual lymphatic drainage is a very light-touch massage designed to help improve the flow of lymph. Excessive lymph that has not drained properly may build up in the soft tissues and cause swelling. This massage is aimed at reducing swelling by redirecting lymph towards the lymph glands, where it can be processed and recirculated.

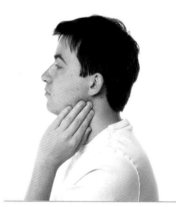
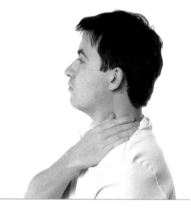

1 Start by treating the neck area, where there are a lot of lymph nodes. Place your hands on either side of your neck with your fingers together, just under the ears. Let your fingers stay still, while you move your arms. Moving your whole arm, trace five very slow circles under your ears.

2 Move your hands down about 2.5 cm/1 in and repeat the technique. Move your hands one or two more times, repeating this same light circular action until you reach the base of the neck. Repeat the whole sequence three to five times.

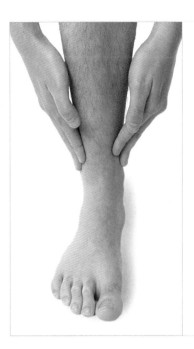

5 Next, move to the area that is swollen. If it is an arm, you will only be able to use one hand at a time; if it is anywhere else on the body, use both hands, as you did for the neck massage. Massage the area in slow, light circles, working in the direction of the lymph flow. Repeat three to five times.

• For the feet, ankles and shins: work towards the knees.
• For the thighs, lower abdomen, hips and lower buttocks: work towards the groin.
• For the lower back: work towards the waist.
• For the upper abdomen, chest and arms: work towards the armpits.
• For the neck and shoulders: work towards the collarbone.
• For the face and head: work towards the jaw or nape of the neck.

Acupressure quick fix

AIMS
to relieve swelling in the lower half of the body

FREQUENCY
three to five times a day

CONTRAINDICATIONS
do not press directly on swollen areas

CROSS-REFERENCE
Knee pain p. 54, Menstrual discomfort p. 60

ALSO BENEFICIAL FOR
knee pain, menstrual cramps

This acupoint is useful for treating swelling in the lower legs and feet.

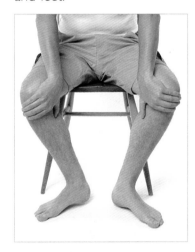

1 Find Spleen 9 by sliding the fingers of your right hand up the inside of your right shinbone. Where the bone runs into the knee, you will feel a curve. Stop here and you should feel a slightly tender area, just under the curve – this is the acupoint.

2 Find the acupoint on the left leg with the left hand and, with both hands, use a circular action to massage the point on both legs. Continue for about two minutes. If possible, elevate your feet afterwards.

Tired feet

Although feet work hard all day, they are often under-appreciated and neglected. Poorly fitting shoes, stifling socks and standing for too long all contribute to sore, aching feet. Because the feet contain so many nerve endings, foot massage can help rejuvenate the entire body. A foot self-massage is a great way to treat yourself at the end of a long day.

Shiatsu self-help

AIMS
to relieve sore feet

FREQUENCY
daily

CONTRAINDICATIONS
do not massage ulcers or open wounds

CROSS-REFERENCE
Energy-boosters p. 40, Pregnancy discomfort p. 68, Stress p. 74

ALSO BENEFICIAL FOR
fatigue, tension, grounding, pregnancy discomfort

If you are flexible enough, sit on the floor with your legs crossed and back supported for this massage. You can also perform it while sitting in a chair.

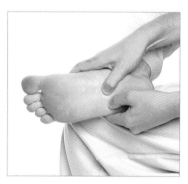

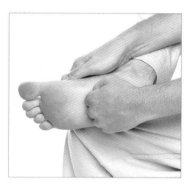

1 *Begin by placing your right foot on your left thigh. With your thumbs together and your fingers wrapped around the top of your foot, press in a straight line from the centre of the heel upwards. Next, use the same technique from the inside of the heel, along the arch, and finally from the outside of your heel up to your last two toes. Repeat the sequence. Each time you press, hold for about one second.*

2 *Next, make a fist with your left hand. Roll the knuckles up the sole, working from the heel to the toes. Repeat this action three or four times.*

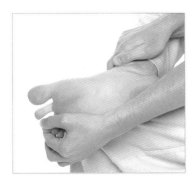

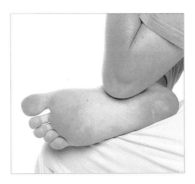

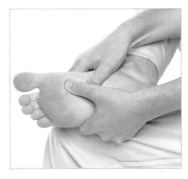

3 *Now take each toe between your thumb and fingers. Roll and squeeze each toe for about 15 seconds.*

4 *If you are flexible enough, take the elbow of your left arm and press it into the sole of your foot. Make small circles with your elbow. After several seconds, move to a different point. Concentrate on the sore areas.*

5 *Finish by squeezing your foot between your fingers and thumbs. Start near the heel, hold for one or two seconds and then move up towards your toes. Repeat the sequence twice. Then repeat it on your left foot.*

Self-massage quick fix

AIMS
to relieve sore feet

FREQUENCY
daily

CONTRAINDICATIONS
do not massage ulcers or open wounds

CROSS-REFERENCE
Energy-boosters p. 40, Pregnancy discomfort p. 68, Stress p. 74

ALSO BENEFICIAL FOR
fatigue, tension, grounding, pregnancy discomfort

This is a technique that is perfect to do while sitting and working at a desk.

1. Use a golf ball under your foot. Press down and roll the ball around with your foot.

2. Make sure you press under the arch and under the toes of the foot.

3. Use your other foot to help hold the golf ball in place.

4. Repeat on the other side.

Toothache

Tooth pain can be caused by cavities or other dental problems. It is important to see your dentist and get the problem corrected professionally. Try these self-massage techniques to help you cope with the pain in the short term, and to recover from dental work.

Reflexology self-help

AIMS
to relieve toothache

FREQUENCY
as needed

CONTRAINDICATIONS
none known

ALSO BENEFICIAL FOR
thyroid imbalances, neck pain

While this reflexology treatment will not cure your toothache, it may give you some temporary relief.

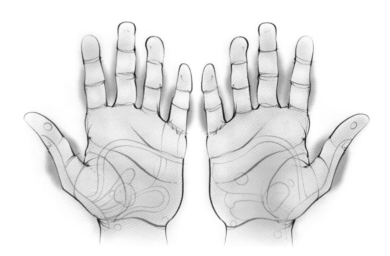

1 *The reflex zone for the teeth is the first knuckle of all the fingers and toes. (see above). Begin by using the index finger and thumb of one hand to stimulate the first knuckle of each finger on the other; also include the first joint of the thumb. Use pinching (see page 20) on the area. Treat each finger for about one minute.*

2 *Next, pinch the first joint of the toes (except the big toe) in the same manner.*

Acupressure quick fix

AIMS
to relieve toothache

FREQUENCY
as needed

CONTRAINDICATIONS
pregnancy

CROSS-REFERENCE
Constipation p. 36,
Headaches p. 46

ALSO BENEFICIAL FOR
constipation, headaches,
facial pain

The well-known acupoint Large Intestine 4 can help relieve toothache. It could also be used to relieve pain experienced after dental work.

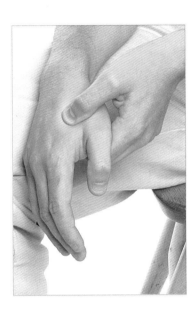

The acupoint Large Intestine 4 is located in the webbing of the thumb and index finger on the back of the hand. To find the point, slide your thumb to where the bones of the index finger and thumb meet, and then press into the bone of the index finger. Press around until you find a tender area.

Massage this point deeply in small circles until the pain lessens.

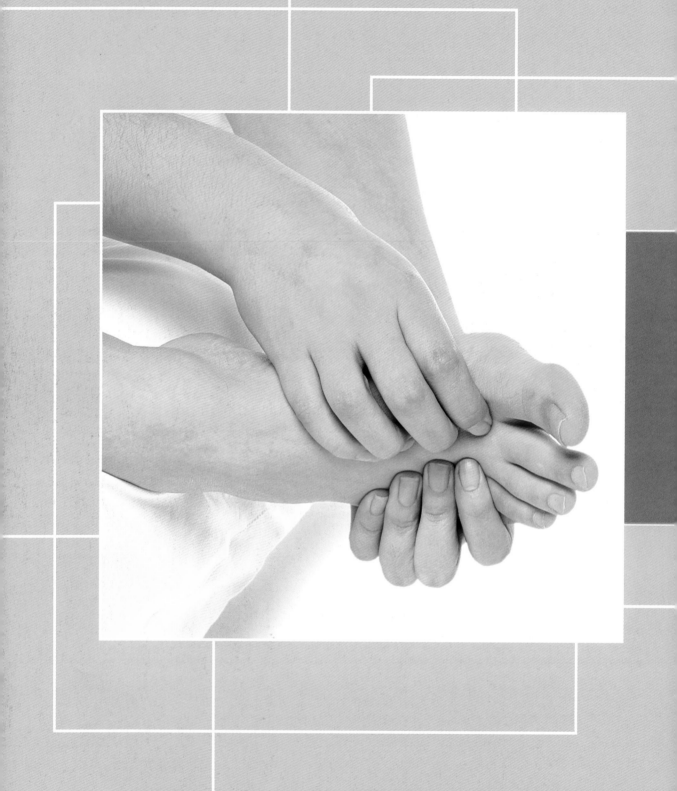

3

WELLNESS ROUTINE

Do-in: *a traditional Asian self-massage*

Do-in is a traditional self-massage from Asia, which relaxes tension, stimulates acupoints, loosens stiff joints and reinvigorates the entire body. Today, many acupressure masters believe that their art developed in ancient times out of the natural tendency to rub and press sore areas of the body. Taoist monks were the first to systematize this self-healing instinct and called their method Tao-Yin ("The Way" or "Gentle approach"). Tao-Yin was considered both a healing tool and a method for promoting general health; the term became "do-in" in Japanese, and today this technique is used as a form of self-help shiatsu.

The aim of this style of self-massage is to harmonize the energy flow through each meridian (a specific channel of energy used in Chinese medicine, see page 18). Do-in helps release toxins, tone the muscles and skin, improve circulation, increase flexibility, reduce aches and pains, and promote self-awareness.

You can do it either standing or sitting. Do-in can be employed as a quick, five-minute re-energizing massage, or as an hour-long healing session, when you work more deeply into the joints, muscles and sore acupoints. It is nice to relax for a while after this massage to allow the effects to settle into your body and mind. You can do this by sitting in a chair and closing your eyes for a few minutes, or by lying down on your back on the floor and resting for around 10 minutes. Follow the sequence set out on pages 87–93, which starts from the head and works down to the feet; or choose parts of the sequence, if you wish to concentrate on a specific area of the body.

Head

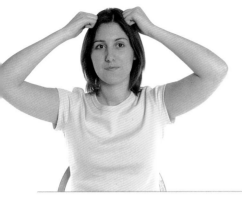 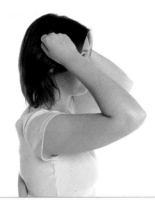 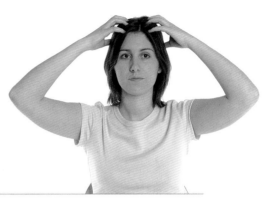

1 *Make fists, but keep your wrists very loose, and tap the top, sides and back of your head.*

2 *Using the same loose fists, tap in circles around each side of the head.*

3 *Use your fingertips to massage from the top of the forehead over the crown of the head and down to the nape of the neck, with a combing and/or circular friction action.*

The face

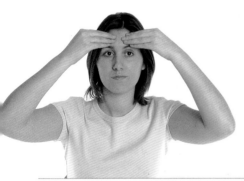 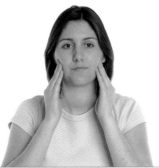 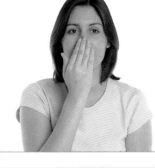

1 *Use your fingertips to massage the forehead with circular friction. Start at the middle and massage outwards to the temples.*

2 *Continue using small circles on the jaw muscles and the cheeks.*

3 *Rub the tip of your nose in a circle using your fingertips.*

4 *Rub and squeeze your ears.*

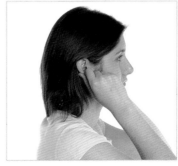

Neck

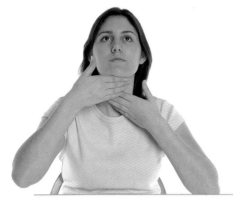 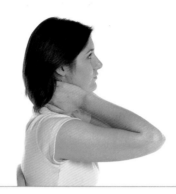 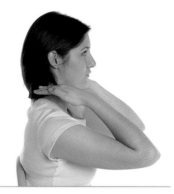

1 Use your fingertips to briskly stroke up the throat.

2 Knead the muscles on the back and sides of the neck.

3 Take a deep breath and, as you exhale, stretch your right ear to the right shoulder, inhale and then stretch your left ear to the left shoulder. Inhale and stretch your chin towards your chest. Inhale and look up, to stretch the front of the throat. Karate-chop the back of your neck from the nape to the shoulders.

Shoulders

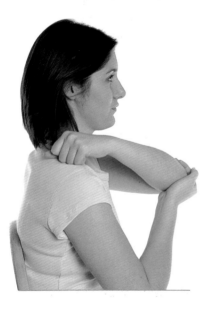

1 Use loose fists to pound the shoulders, using the right hand on the left shoulder and vice versa.

2 Grasp and knead the area from the base of your neck out to the shoulder joint. Repeat on the other side.

3 Circle your shoulders back and forwards several times.

4 Inhale, draw your shoulders up to your ears, exhale strongly and throw your shoulders back down in a shrug. Repeat three times.

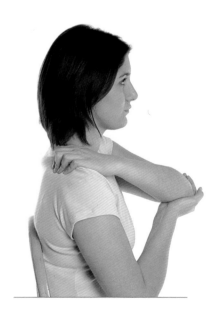

Hands and arms

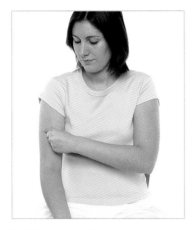

1 Use a loose fist to tap down the inside of the arm (from the upper arm to the palm of the hand) and up the outside of the arm. Repeat three times.

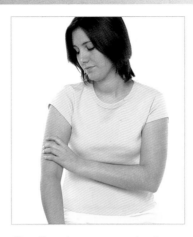

2 Knead, squeeze and twist the muscles of your arm, from just below the armpit to the hand.

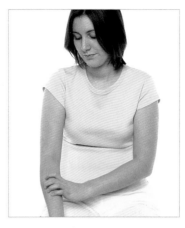

3 Briskly brush down your arm.

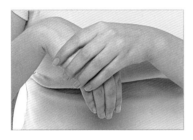

4 Stretch your wrist in both directions.

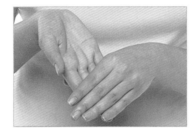

5 Gently pulling your fingers down will help to stretch the wrist.

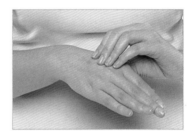

6 Use your fingertips to massage the spaces between the bones of the hand.

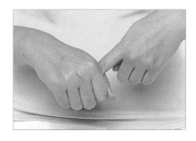

7 Squeeze and twist each finger and the thumb from the base to the tip.

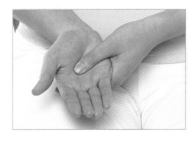

8 Use your thumb to massage the palm of the hand.

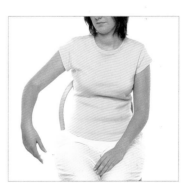

9 Give your whole arm a shake. Repeat on the other hand.

Torso

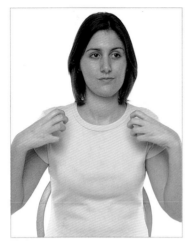

1 Bend your fingers and make them firm. Use the tips of your fingers to quickly tap the front of the ribcage while taking a deep breath.

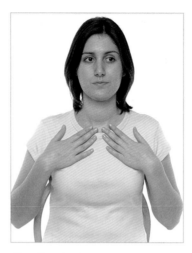

2 Exhale through your mouth and repeatedly slap the ribs using your whole palm. Repeat three times.

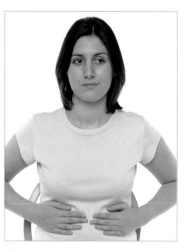

3 Repeat this step on the sides of the ribs.

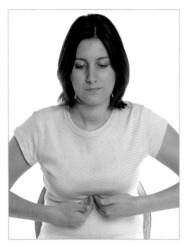

4 Bring your fingers just under the ribcage. Take a deep breath and, as you exhale, bend forward and massage deep into the abdomen with your fingertips. Repeat three to five times, moving your fingers to a slightly different place on the abdomen each time.

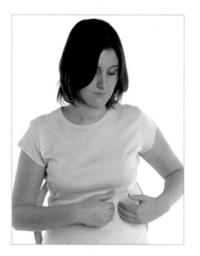

5 Use all of your fingertips together to make small circles on your abdomen. Begin just under your breastbone, as if this was 12 o'clock. Massage for about 15 seconds. Next move

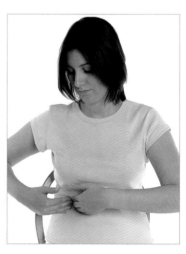

your fingertips to one o'clock and massage in small circles again. Continue until you're back at 12 o'clock. Now reverse the direction for 12 more circles.

Back

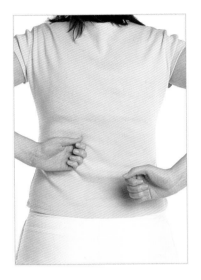

Make loose fists with your hands. Tap your lower back, from the ribs down towards your tailbone. Then tap your tailbone and your buttocks.

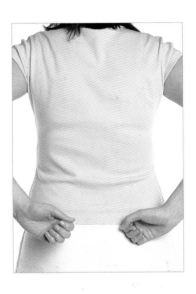

2 Place your hands on your waist, with your fingers wrapped around the front and your thumbs to the back. Move your thumbs to the muscles along the spine. Lean back as you press your thumbs into and massage these muscles. Move your thumbs down a little further and repeat.

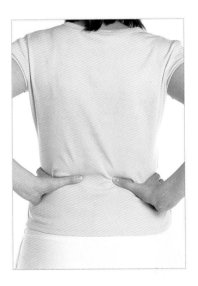

Legs and feet

You can do this section sitting in a chair or on the floor.

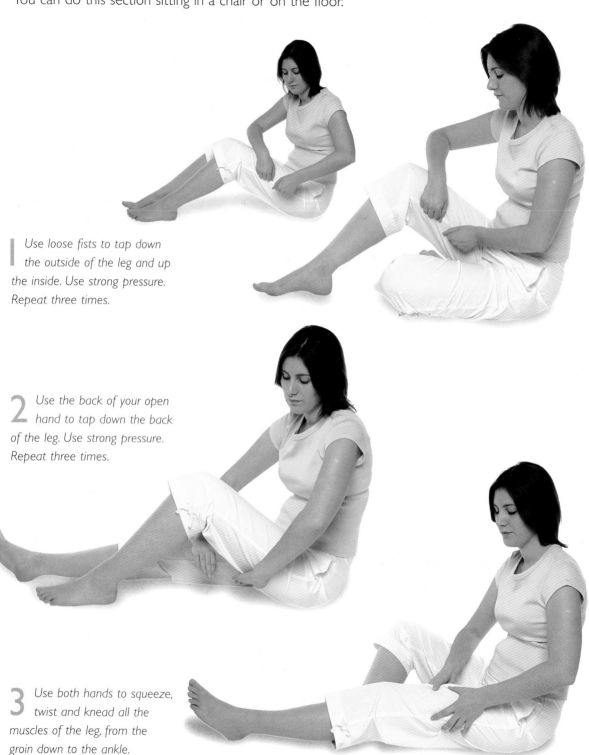

1 Use loose fists to tap down the outside of the leg and up the inside. Use strong pressure. Repeat three times.

2 Use the back of your open hand to tap down the back of the leg. Use strong pressure. Repeat three times.

3 Use both hands to squeeze, twist and knead all the muscles of the leg, from the groin down to the ankle.

Legs and feet continued

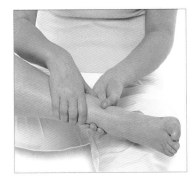

4 Place one foot on top of your thigh, to work on the foot. (Sit in a chair if necessary.) Grasp the ankle with both hands and shake your foot vigorously.

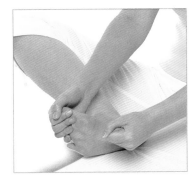

5 Stretch your toes back and use a loose fist on the opposite hand to tap the sole of the foot.

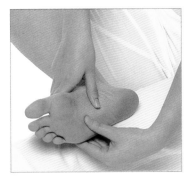

6 Use the thumbs to massage the sole of the foot.

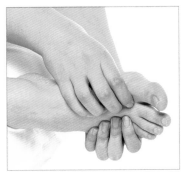

7 Use the fingertips to massage the spaces between the bones on top of the foot.

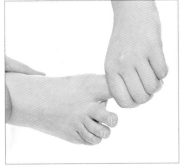

8 Massage and twist each toe.

9 Gently bounce your whole leg. Repeat the whole sequence on the other leg. Now relax for 5–10 minutes, either lying on the floor or reclining in a chair with your eyes closed. Breathe deeply and allow the abdomen to rise and fall with each breath. When you are ready, open your eyes, get up and notice the positive shift in your energy!

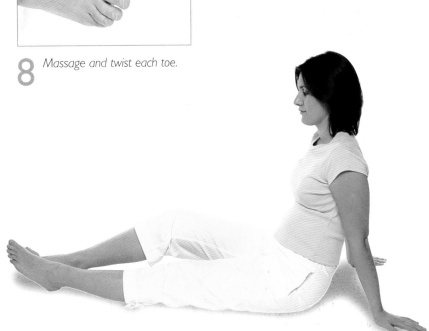

index

bibliography/acknowledgments

General Massage

Davies, Clair, *The Trigger Point Therapy Workbook*. Oakland, CA: New Harbinger Publications, Inc. (2001)

Maxwell-Hudson, Clare, *Complete Massage: A Visual Guide to Over 100 Techniques*. New York: DK Publishing Inc. (2001)

Acupressure and Chinese Medicine

Gach, Michael Reed, *Acupressure's Potent Points: A Guide to Self-Care for Common Ailments*, New York: Bantam Books (1990).

Maciocia, Giovanni, *The Foundations of Chinese Medicine: A Comprehensive Text for Acupuncturists and Herbalists*, Edinburgh: Churchill Livingstone (1989)

Shen, Peijian, *Massage for Pain Relief: A Step-by-Step Guide*, New York: Random House (1996)

Reflexology

Dougans, Inge with Ellis, Suzanne, *The Art of Reflexology: A Step-by-Step Guide*, Rockport: MA Element Books Inc. (1992)

Kunz, Kevin and Barbara, *Hand and Foot Reflexology: A Self-Help Guide*, New York: Fireside (1992)

Indian Head Massage

Brown, Denise Whichello, *Teach Yourself: Indian Head Massage*, Chicago: Contemporary Books (2003)

Chrysalis Books Group Plc is committed to respecting the intellectual property rights of others. We have therefore taken all reasonable efforts to ensure that the reproduction of all content on these pages is done with the full consent of copyright owners. If you are aware of any unintentional ommissions please contact the company directly so that any necessary corrections may be made for future editions.

All photographs shot by Neil Sutherland, except:
p 6 Mary Evans Picture Library
p 7 Werner Forman Archive

Artwork by Juliet Percival

I'd like to thank my teachers: Michael Reed Gach and the instructors at the Acupressure Institute in California, and Saul Goodman and the instructors at the International School of Shiatsu in Pennsylvania. Thanks to Rene Stephens, Valerie Hartman and Genie Hardee for reading the manuscript and offering their suggestions and expertise. I'd also like to thank Jane Ellis at Chrysalis books for her patient and methodical organizing and editing, and Juliet Percival for her beautiful artwork. A special thanks to my dear friend Martina Barnes for her love, support and encouragement. Finally, thanks to my husband Bhavesh and my baby boy Bhaerava for creating the space in our lives for this book to come into being.

Kristine Kaoverii Weber

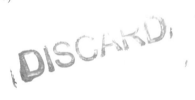